What is PSORIASIS ?

All About Psoriasis for Psoriasis Patients

Dean R. Goodless, M.D.

What is Psoriasis?

© 2012 New Paradigm Dermatology, PL

ISBN-13:
978-1475132823

ISBN-10:
1475132824

First Printing, 2012

Printed in the United States of America

What is Psoriasis?

What is Psoriasis?

About the Author:

Dr. Goodless is a board-certified dermatologist and a fellow of the American Academy of Dermatology. He is in private practice in the Orlando, Fla. area.

Experience:

With 20 years of clinical experience treating psoriasis, Dr. Goodless has had the opportunity to use every treatment available for this common, but troublesome disease. He has served as principle or sub-investigator on over a dozen FDA clinical drug trials, including several for new psoriasis drugs.

Education:

Dr. Goodless received his medical degree from the University of Miami. Postgraduate training included an internship at University of Florida and a second year of internal medicine residency at Mt. Sinai Medical Center in Miami Beach. He completed his dermatology training in the three-year dermatology residency program at University of Miami School of Medicine and was subsequently certified by the American Board of Dermatology.

From Dr. Goodless, M.D.:

Psoriasis can be frustrating to manage, but you are not alone. Some 2% of people suffer from psoriasis, millions in the United States alone. I hope that my experience and insight will assist you in understanding psoriasis, as well as the treatment options available for this disease. Finally, I'm not just a dispassionate observer in regards to psoriasis. Like you...I am also a psoriasis patient.

What is Psoriasis?

Contents

What is Psoriasis?

Section One

What is Psoriasis?

Answer:
Psoriasis is a chronic skin condition usually resulting in thickening of the skin with associated redness and scaling. Its appearance can vary depending upon which part of the skin is involved. Thick, scaly, red plaques are the hallmark of psoriasis. In psoriatic skin, the cells of the outer layer (epidermis) multiply too rapidly, which causes skin to thicken. They also adhere to one another more strongly and for longer than normal skin cells do, resulting in scaliness. The skin is infiltrated by white blood cells, causing inflammation, redness, and rarely pustules. Why this happens is not well known, but genetics are clearly involved.

People of any age can get psoriasis. It can be detected on the skin of infants before they're even born or can appear for the first time in those well into their senior years. Most patients first get the disease either in early adult life or when they're in their fifties. Some with psoriasis have the disease throughout their lifetime, although the severity can range from barely noticeable to hard to ignore. Certain factors can worsen psoriasis, including medications and skin trauma.

Psoriasis is not infectious and cannot be passed directly from one person to another. Although very rapid growth of skin cells is seen in psoriasis, it is still a benign process and not related cancer.

1

What Causes Psoriasis?

The exact underlying cause of psoriasis is not fully known. However, there are certain known contributing factors that strongly support theories about the disease. Sparing the advanced biochemistry: Researchers know that there are processes going on in your body that lead to increased inflammation, and therefore thickening of the skin and scaliness. What is less well understood, however, is *why* this happens in the first place.

Heredity plays a strong role in psoriasis, especially in those who develop it early on. The majority of these people report having a sibling or other family member who has psoriasis as well. That said, one might assume that identical twins would both have psoriasis if it was in their genetic cards. But this is not always the case, meaning that there is likely an environmental influence that factors in, too.

Many diseases (including psoriasis) have been linked to specific HLA types, which are genetically encoded into our DNA. These HLA types produce markers that appear on the surface of white blood cells and that can be easily determined with routine lab tests. Different groups of psoriasis patients seem to be more likely to carry a few specific types of genetic HLA associations. In one group, psoriasis that appears early in life as well as in another family member is common. In another, those with psoriasis don't develop it until they're in their fifties and none of their relatives have it.

Keeping in mind these two very different groups, it becomes clearer to see that it is likely that several different genes – including so called "psoriasis susceptibility and severity genes" – play a role in this complex disease.

What is Psoriasis?

Still, environmental and other trigger factors seem to play a role in the severity or onset of the disease, too. For example, some patients may have a psoriasis breakout after suffering a strep throat infection. Surgical cuts or wounds may turn into psoriasis (a phenomenon known as *Koebnerization*) in certain people. Many medications are even associated with causing or worsening psoriasis. Stress, although overemphasized as a factor in most psoriasis cases, may play in role in select patients. Some accountants may see a worsening of their psoriasis around tax season, for example, while others may not.

Misconceptions About Psoriasis

As someone who treats psoriasis, I frequently have patients who bring common mis-understandings about the condition to my attention. Here are just a few common myths about psoriasis that need debunking:

- **Psoriasis is contagious**
  You can not pass the disease onto others, for example, by touching them. Psoriasis is genetic, though flare-ups or worsening of the condition may occur as a result of infections, such as strep throat.
- **Psoriasis is cancer**
  Psoriasis causes skin cells to grow rapidly, but the condition is not in any way related to skin cancer. There may be a very slight increased risk of lymphoma in psoriasis patients (2%) compared to the general population (1%).
- **Psoriasis is due to "dirty" blood**
  While there are definitely increased compounds, such as TNF alpha, in the blood of those with psoriasis, these are not waste products or contaminants to be removed or filtered – they are natural compounds that

should be present. Psoriasis has nothing to do with "contaminated" blood.

- **"Nobody in my family has psoriasis, therefore I can't have psoriasis."**
  Psoriasis is very common, affecting roughly 2% of the population. While many patients can recall a relative with the condition, some do not. This does not "rule out" psoriasis. You may have a relative whose psoriasis is hidden, or you may have a relative who had the condition, but has since passed on.
- **There is a "secret cure" for psoriasis**
  Maybe a friend, relative, or website mentioned a "100% effective and completely safe" psoriasis treatment – I really wish this were true! It's nice to think that there is a one shot deal that will permanently make that rash go away, but it – unfortunately – doesn't exist.

Diagnosis and Evaluation of Psoriasis

What Does Your Doctor Look for?

A Straightforward Diagnosis – Most of the Time
Psoriasis is usually an easy thing for most dermatologists to diagnose. That is, it can typically be diagnosed on sight based on skin changes and the location of the condition on the body. No further testing is needed unless there is some confusion about the diagnosis. For example, a physician may find it more difficult to diagnose a patient who also has another condition, such as eczema. In these rare instances, a skin biopsy is usually easily able to make a specific diagnosis.

What is Psoriasis?

Just How Bad is it?
Somewhat more complicated than diagnosing psoriasis is evaluating how severe it is. How much of the body is covered? How severe is the rash in those areas? What is the effect on the patient's quality of life?

To answer these questions, objective measures have been developed to help compare one patient to another, or to assess a given patient's condition over time. More often than not, these more sophisticated measurements are used in clinical trials. However, they may be used in a doctor's office to justify a certain treatment for a patient, especially newer biologic agents, which can be very expensive. In these instances, insurance companies often require some sort of objective evidence that a patient's psoriasis is severe enough to warrant the expense of these drugs.

An Objective Measurement
The most commonly used "objective measure" is the Psoriasis Area Severity Index, also known as the PASI score. The body is divided into four areas – head, trunk, upper extremities and lower extremities – each of which carries a different weight based on the percentage of body surface they represent. Each area is assessed separately for the severity of psoriasis, specifically thickness, redness and scaliness. After a little bit of mathematics, a score is assigned from 0 to 72. Following this score over time is sometimes useful to assess a response to a particular treatment. More often, this is used during clinical trials of new treatments to prove effectiveness.

A Newer Way of Looking at Psoriasis Severity
A newer measurement called the Koo-Menter Psoriasis Instrument is a questionnaire that can be used to assess the effect that psoriasis has on a patient's overall quality of life.

What is Psoriasis?

Insurance companies are now taking a closer look at this sort of subjective measure, since a patient with a relatively low PASI score may still have severe quality of life issues if the areas involved interfere with daily activities or have tremendous social implications (such as the face, hands or genitals). In these instances, the Koo-Menter Psoriasis Instrument may give a more accurate portrayal of the severity of a patient's psoriasis.

Symptoms of Psoriasis

More than just a skin rash

Identifying psoriasis requires looking for characteristic skin changes which in many instances have a predilection for specific body parts. Thickening of skin, scaling and redness are all typical changes seen in psoriatic skin. Additionally, psoriasis can affect *not just skin*, but nails, scalp, and joints as well. In other words, psoriasis has findings typical for both *what* and *where*. Key features of Psoriasis include:

What: Skin Plaques

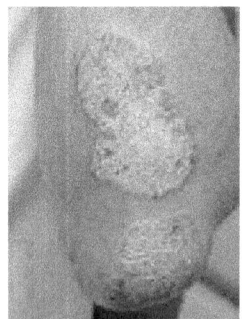
©*New Paradigm Dermatology, PL*

Plaque-type psoriasis is the most common form of the disease, hence the name *psoriasis vulgaris*. The three hallmarks of a plaque of psoriasis are: thickened skin, red skin and skin scales. The thickness of a plaque (a raised skin lesion more

All About Psoriasis for Psoriasis Patients Page 6

What is Psoriasis?

than 1cm in diameter which can be felt) can vary from barely perceptible to several millimeters thick. They range in color from a faint pink to deep beefy red. In patients with darker skin types, there may be less redness and more darkening of the skin. Scales can range from virtually absent to thick oyster-shell like adherent plates known as ostraceous scales.

What: Auspitz's Sign
When adherent psoriatic scales are scraped or picked off, pinpoint bleeding known as Auspitz's sign may occur. The pinpoint areas represent the tops of tiny capillaries which undulate vertically throughout the thickened psoriatic skin.

What: Koebner Phenomenon
The Koebner phenomenon (Koebnerization, isomorphic response) occurs when a new area of psoriasis develops in injured skin. For example, after a surgery, psoriasis may develop around the surgical scar. This phenomenon may also help explain why psoriasis tends to occur on areas of constant low-intensity trauma such as elbows and knees. Koebnerization can occur after non-traumatic skin injury such as a sunburn, or an allergic reaction to a medication. In patients who suffer from dandruff or seborrheic dermatitis of the face and scalp, psoriasis can superimpose itself due to irritation and scratching and a crossover or combination dermatitis known as "sebopsoriasis" develops. Koebnerization is not specific to psoriasis.

What: Guttate, Pustular and Erythrodermic Psoriasis
These less common forms of psoriasis differ dramatically from the typical plaque type. In Guttate (drop-like) psoriasis, tiny papules (lesions which can be felt and are less than 1cm in diameter) appear sprinkled throughout the skin. Pustular psoriasis can occur in smaller areas or involve most of the

What is Psoriasis?

body with innumerable tiny white pustules. Eythrodermic Psoriasis occurs when the entire body turns bright red and scaly. In this instance, a skin biopsy may be needed to separate erythrodermic psoriasis from other diseases which also can cause a universally red and scaly skin (known as *exfoliative erythroderma* or "red man").

Where: Typical Locations

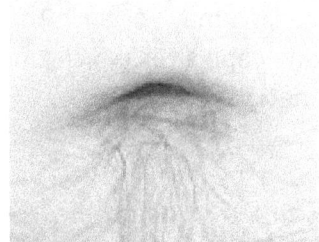

© *New Paradigm Dermatolog, PL*

Plaque type psoriasis typically involves specific locations on the body including the scalp, elbow, knees, genitals, belly button (umbilicus) and buttocks area (sacrum and intergluteal cleft). In damp areas such as the armpits, under breasts or in the groin, scales become macerated (wet and pasty) and the lesions take on a moist, red and raw appearance closely mimicking a yeast infection in appearance. On the scalp, a severe form of dandruff-like flaking and scaling can be seen.

Where: Hand and Foot Lesions

Psoriasis of the hands and feet can have either a plaque like appearance as seen in other body areas, or a pustular appearance. The presence of pustules is usually attributed to infections, however in psoriasis, pustules form as a part of the inflammatory response. Very thickened plaques on the palms or soles, being somewhat inflexible, may crack with movement. The resulting fissures can be painful and sometimes become secondarily infected. Severe foot lesions can result in disability by limiting your ability to walk.

Where: Finger and Toenails

Nail changes commonly seen in psoriasis include thickening, lifting, and pitting of the nails. "Oil spotting" (darkened areas where the nail appears translucent similar to the effect of placing a drop of oil on a sheet of paper) are fairly specific for this disease. Treatment of nail psoriasis can be difficult.

Where: Joints (Psoriatic Arthritis)

Psoriatic arthritis is an inflammatory arthritis which can affect up to 10% of patients with moderate to severe psoriasis. Five distinct patterns of arthritis occur in psoriasis which can sometimes be separated from rheumatoid arthritis by x-ray findings or blood tests.

Treating it Yourself: Things You Can Try Before You See Your Doctor

Natural sunlight or *heliotherapy* is a potent psoriasis treatment. Exposure to sunlight, without burning, is sometimes able to clear patients completely. Many of my own patients make it a habit to get to the beach every few weeks to keep their skin clear. Meditation has been shown to help speed up the rate at which phototherapy (artificial sunlight) can clear psoriasis. A healthy diet is good for you and good for your skin. Fresh fruits and veggies or even a gluten-free diet may be useful. Avoid those things known to cause or flare psoriasis including smoking, alcohol, obesity, certain medications, and minor skin trauma.

What is Psoriasis?

There are a few OTC topical medications which may help pso-riasis. Many of these are coal tar derivatives, which have a distinctive odor. Coal tar products can increase the sensitivity of the skin to sunlight and cause a sunburn in those unaware of this. On the other hand, coal tar medication applied careful-ly directly to psoriasis plaques an hour or so before natural sun exposure is also a potent treatment in and of itself.

Topical corticosteroids in OTC creams are limited to hydrocor-tisone 1%. Although somewhat weak, this strength of hydrocortisone can sometimes be quite effective for psoriasis of the face, armpits or groin. It's just too weak to treat thicker plaques on the elbows, knees, hands and feet however.

Finally, good 'ol petroleum jelly has been shown to be some-what helpful in treating psoriasis – just be prepared for a little bit of a mess.

Heliotherapy: Nature's Treatment for Psoriasis

Effective, Yes – But Read the Fine Print First
Natural sunlight contains many wavelengths of light besides visible light: invisible ultraviolet radiation is present as well. Ultraviolet radiation is often used to treat psoriasis in the doc-tor's office using special equipment. Heliotherapy (also called climatotherapy) makes simple use of intentional direct expo-sure to natural sunlight to get the therapeutic benefits of the included ultraviolet radiation.

The use of heliotherapy began a long time ago when it was used in India, China and Egypt to treat diseases, including pso-riasis. Ancient Greeks also used natural sunlight as therapy. As far back as 3,000 years, medical practitioners were advanced enough to use sunlight-sensitizing chemicals before sun expo-sure – a primitive version of today's photochemotherapy or PUVA. Heliotherapy has been studied, and it works. Benefits lasting beyond a year have even been documented.

Words of Caution
The same invisible ultraviolet radiation that treats psoriasis is also responsible for many undesirable skin changes as well. These same wavelengths of light can also cause skin aging, wrinkling, tanning, burning and skin cancer. For this reason, heliotherapy should be applied with the same caution, fore-thought and examination of risks, benefits, and alternatives as any other psoriasis therapy.

Heliotherapy should be avoided by anyone with a history of alcoholism or serious mental health issues, as well as those taking photosensitizing medications. Careful exposure to noonday sun – for short periods at first, and longer periods as tolerated – should give significant results in as little as 3 to 4 weeks. Inform your physician if you plan to use heliotherapy to be certain that it will not conflict with any of your other medications. For those willing to travel for a supervised course of heliotherapy, spas at the Dead Sea in Israel offer what is generally considered the ultimate heliotherapy experience.

Meditation and Psoriasis

Put Your Mind to it
Psoriasis, like many disorders involving the immune system, is somewhat effected by emotional stress. Some people with psoriasis report that their psoriasis first appeared or worsened after a stressful life event.

What is Psoriasis?

Mindfulness meditation to reduce stress can be beneficial in psoriasis. In one study, published in the journal *Psychosomatic Medicine*, people with psoriasis were treated with ultraviolet light therapy. Some received their treatments while listening to meditation tapes, others received just the light. Patients receiving both cleared their psoriasis up to 4 times faster.

Will Changing Your Diet Help Your Psoriasis?

It is clear that what we eat has a tremendous impact on our overall health. Less clear is the question of modifying our diets to actually treat an ongoing disease such as Psoriasis.

Current Status

The most promising role for dietary manipulation in the treatment of psoriasis involves following a gluten-free diet. Gluten is a storage protein / starch compound found in grasses such as wheat, rye and barley. Some people have antibodies to one component of gluten called gliadin resulting in a condition known as celiac disease. When these people eat bread and other gluten-containing foods they may get gastrointestinal symptoms and break out in a pustular skin eruption called *dermatitis herpetiformis*. Pustules can also be seen in certain types of psoriasis, and more people with psoriasis have anti-gliadin antibodies than the general population. Although the data is small at present, there are some studies and dramatic case reports showing improvement in psoriasis with the adoption of a gluten-free diet. A similar condition called *palmo-plantar pustulosis* (which some argue is a variant of psoriasis) also improves on this type of diet.

Background

In general, the paths that "suggestive" dietary studies have lead researchers down have typically ended in disappointment. One promising idea was that fish oil would benefit those with Psoriasis. It seems that Greenland Eskimos have relatively less psoriasis and rheumatoid arthritis and it was believed that diet played a role by providing more of the anti-inflammatory omega-3 fish oils. Indeed, when these people immigrated to Denmark and took on a diet which included much more red meat, they developed psoriasis and arthritis at a significantly higher rate. Unfortunately, studies supplementing fish oil into the diet of patients with psoriasis have been relatively disappointing. Greenland Eskimos it seems are equipped with a genetic advantage allowing them to make use of the fish oil to reduce the onset of inflammatory diseases. In the absence of this genetic background, most psoriasis patients see no benefit in their skin from the use of Omega-3 supplements.

Miscellaneous studies have shown some slight benefits from what would appear to be simply *healthy eating*: fresh fruits and vegetables, small amounts of protein from fish and fowl, fiber supplements, olive oil, and avoidance of red meat, processed foods, and refined carbohydrates. One study found psoriasis to be inversely associated with intake of carrots, tomatoes, and fresh fruit.

Should You Try This?
There are certainly many good reasons supporting eating a healthy diet laden with fresh fruits and vegetables. Other than eating right, large changes in diet will probably be unrewarding.

Gluten-Free Diet for All?
In fact, psoriasis patients only have a marginally higher incidence of anti-gliadin antibodies than others. In the absence of these antibodies, following a strict gluten-free diet would not

only be useless in improving psoriasis, but would mean giving up most traditional breads, pastas, and cereals permanently.

Where it Stands

Eat a healthy diet with lots of fresh fruits and vegetables, minimize red meats and if you doctor thinks it would be helpful, check for anti-gliadin antibodies.

Do I Need to See a Doctor About My Psoriasis?

Answer: You may. There are certain times when you should get the help of a knowledgeable doctor (preferably a board certified dermatologist) instead of trying to treat your skin yourself. Does your psoriasis...

- cover a good portion of your body (10% or more)?
- involve your face, hands or genitalia?
- involve very thick or scaly plaques that over-the-counter medicines have been unable to help?
- seem to have suddenly worsened? (redness all over your body, or the development of white, pus-filled lesions)
- accompany joint pain and/or swelling?
- seem unresponsive to all the self-directed treatments you've already tried?

If you've answered "yes" to one or more of these questions, your psoriasis is likely to be severe enough to need a prescription medication. Please see your dermatologist.

Finding the Right Doctor for Your Psoriasis

You may wonder which doctor you should see to treat your psoriasis. Most primary care physicians have some experience with psoriasis and can easily manage a simple case, which requires only topical treatment of small areas. What do you do when your whole body is covered or when you have painful psoriatic arthritis associated with your psoriasis, though? What type of doctor is well-versed in the use of biologic drugs, methotrexate and other strong medicines?

When your psoriasis reaches a point where your primary care physician is no longer comfortable treating you, ask to be referred to a qualified dermatologist in your community. A dermatologist is a physician who has completed specialized training in skin diseases after completing medical school. For most MDs, this means three years of intensive hospital-based training. Many dermatologists treat the full spectrum of skin diseases, but there are also centers dedicated to psoriasis treatment.

For those patients with severe psoriatic arthritis who are not responsive to their dermatologist's treatment, referral to a rheumatologist may be useful. Rheumatologists specialize in the treatment of arthritis and may have access to intravenous medications, such as Remicade, while most dermatologists do not.

Finding a qualified dermatologist is as easy as visiting the website for the American Academy of Dermatology (AAD). Fellows of the AAD have completed a dermatology residency and passed the examination of the American Board of Dermatology. Their website URL is www.AAD.org.

What is Psoriasis?

Your Doctor and Your Psoriasis

Know a bit about treatment options for psoriasis in general. You don't have to know the names of medications, but you should be aware of the different treatment options that your doctor may offer so that you can be active in the decision making process. Possible treatments include:

- topical creams
- phototherapy or treatment with ultraviolet light
- systemic pills
- systemic injections

You may have already decided some of these are not for you. For example, can you spare the time for the three office visits per week that phototherapy entails? Are you so afraid of needles that you can't imagine giving yourself an injection which is needed for some biologic therapies?

Sometimes your past medical or social history is critical in deciding what treatments you should take. For example, a patient with liver disease or who is actively drinking alcohol shouldn't take Methotrexate for their psoriasis. Those with a personal or family history of multiple sclerosis may wish to avoid Enteracept. Your doctor needs to know all about you before prescribing many of the drugs used in psoriasis.

Some of your existing medications may conflict with your psoriasis treatment. For example many medications make you sensitive to sunlight, making phototherapy problematic. Your doctor needs a complete list of all your current medications. Finally, he will need to know any drugs you are allergic to.

What is Psoriasis?

Psoriasis treatment can be very expensive depending upon the medications needed. Your doctor can work within your budget, or sometimes get assistance for more expensive drugs directly from the manufacturers. My office is always well stocked with coupons from drug manufacturers designed to help patients with their part of the bill at the pharmacy – it may be worth asking your doctor if any such discounts are available. Some of the biologic companies will give away their medicines to qualified patients. Insurance companies often use seemingly arbitrary and capricious rules to decide which medications they are willing to pay for, but sometimes with a flurry of letters and appeals they will cover drugs they initially deny payment for.

If you drink, fess up. Alcohol and Methotrexate is a dangerous combination. Do you have psoriasis in a sensitive area, such as the genitals? Don't assume the cream given for your elbows and knees will be safe if used elsewhere. For areas such as the armpits, groin and under the breasts, strong steroid creams can cause side effects such as stretch marks and thinning of the skin (which can be permanent). Don't be embarrassed to speak with your doctor about this – doctors have dealt with these concerns before and want to ensure that you are safe during treatment. If you need a treatment for a specific area, it's best to speak up.

Will My Children Get Psoriasis?

Answer: Many parents with psoriasis wonder if their children will also get the disease. Since psoriasis has a genetic basis, the question is legitimate, but the answers are often estimates at best. Psoriasis has a genetic basis: Thirty-six percent to 91% of patients have some sort of family history of the disease. If both parents and a sibling have psoriasis however, the risk is as high as 83. Here are some other statistics to consider:

- one sibling with psoriasis: risk is 24%
- one parent with psoriasis: risk is 28%
- one sibling and one parent with psoriasis: risk is 41%
- two parents with psoriasis: risk is 65%

Note that in no case is the risk 100%, meaning that no one can say for certain that a given child will have psoriasis no matter what the family history. Also realize that *psoriasis can occur in the complete absence of any family history.*

A Historical Look at Psoriasis

From the Perspective of Dr. Von Hebra – the First "Official" Dermatologist

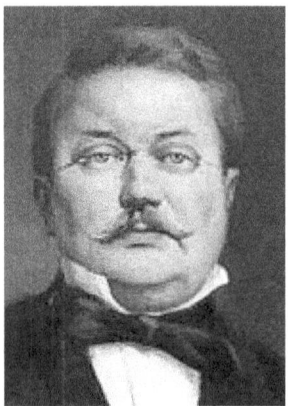

Dr. Ferdinand Ritter Von Hebra (*public domain*)

Some 20 years ago, I picked up a little treasure at our medical school library's book sale: *Von Hebra on: Diseases of the Skin* (1867). While it is of little other than historical value at pre-

What is Psoriasis?

sent, I thought it might be entertaining to take a look at the chapter on psoriasis.

Von Hebra was the head of what is ostensibly considered the first "official" department of dermatology at the University of Vienna. More than any other modern dermatologist, he is responsible for naming and categorizing the dermatology lexicon still in use today.

By researching literature of the ancient Greeks, Egyptians and medieval scholars, he separated out the many diseases confused and lumped together with psoriasis into their proper categories. The disease he describes and categorized as psoriasis is in fact the disease we consider as psoriasis today.

Many people wonder why psoriasis has such a strange sounding name, but it's certainly much less of a tongue twister than *Dartre squameuse centrifuge of Alibert* another name for this disease laid to rest by the esteemed professor (thank you Dr. Von Hebra).

Among the causes of psoriasis Von Hebra lists climatic conditions, habits (including brandy) and nervous temperaments. Not too far off the mark from what we understand today (genetics was not yet considered). He claims to have treated more than 1,000 patients with psoriasis and found that, in general, they were overall healthy and free from other significant illness, and that no particular occupation predisposed people to the condition. These findings were somewhat divergent from his contemporaries of the day.

Treatment-wise, Von Hebra was not very happy with the various medications of the day which he claimed tended to cause "violent reactions." Instead he preferred to use arsenicals (medications derived from arsenic). Although these medicines did work and were employed for a variety of ailments, they are obviously much too toxic to be considered as a medical treatment for any disease today. Tar preparations were also a part of his treatment armamentarium. It makes you wonder: What will doctors 100 years from now say about our current treatments?

That concludes this brief look at psoriasis from a historical perspective. From a practical point of view, the most important thing to glean from Von Hebra might be to look at treatments with a somewhat cynical view – to not just accept historical or anecdotal evidence as a means of establishing whether or not a treatment is useful, but to use scientific observation.

Why Is Psoriasis Called Psoriasis?

Answer:
It was Dr. Ferdinand Ritter Von Hebra who first used the term psoriasis in 1841 to describe this disease. Von Hebra was a dermatologist at the University of Vienna. He was the first doctor to study skin diseases from the viewpoint of anatomical pathology. In other words, he studied various skin diseases under the microscope and categorized them according to their microscopic features. This meticulous approach cleared up much confusion about the causes and nature of various skin diseases, many of which looked similar to the naked eye. Von Hebra's work remains a foundation upon which we continue our understanding of skin diseases. Of course, we now have new tools at our disposal – including molecular and genetic studies – which he could only dream of.

The term *psoro* comes from the Greek word for itch; *psoriasis* corresponds with the term *itchy*. The term *psoriasis* was used as early as 1684 as the Latin term for mange. Mange is simply another word for scabies, a very itchy mite infestation (which, in fact, has no relation to psoriasis).

Von Hebra used the term psoriasis to describe the disease we all know today as psoriasis. Once his system of skin classifications became the standard, all other names for this disease were relegated to historical status.

Pustular Psoriasis

In pustular psoriasis, the skin will develop pus-filled lesions called pustules. Although pustules are typically associated with infection, in pustular psoriasis the lesions are formed as the result of inflammation, usually in the absence of infection. Both *generalized* and *localized* types of pustular psoriasis are recognized.

Generalized Pustular Psoriasis
Generalized pustular psoriasis (GPP) has four recognized patterns:
- von Zumbusch pattern: a whole-body painful eruption accompanied by systemic symptoms such as fever and malaise. Innumerable pustules form which can sometimes come together into larger "lakes of pus".
- Annular pattern: growing and spreading rings with an advancing edge of pustules. The lesions enlarge and spread over hours to days with central clearing. Systemic symptoms may again be seen.
- Exanthematic type: This is usually an abrupt eruption of tiny pustules, typically without systemic symptoms and with relatively rapid clearing. This may be a type of drug eruption when associated with a medication such as lithium. I have also seen this happen more than

once with Ciprofloxacin. Another name for this rash in the setting of a drug eruption is *acute generalized exanthematous pustulosis*.

- "Localized" pattern: In patients with widespread plaque type psoriasis, pustules may develop within or at the edges of plaques. This can be seen with irritating treatments such as coal tar or even rapid withdrawal of potent topical steroids.

Localized types of pustular psoriasis

Pustular psoriasis can be limited to the palms and soles or just the fingertips/ends of toes. When the palms and soles are involved, the condition is sometimes termed *palmoplantar pustulosis*. Fintertip pustular psoriasis, called *Acrodermatitis continua of Hallopeau* can be accompanied by complete shedding of the nails.

How to Avoid Pustular Psoriasis

Several factors have been known to increase the risk of the various types of pustular psoriasis and avoiding or minimizing these may be helpful:

- Avoid systemic corticosteroids like injections or oral prednisone for treating psoriasis
- Avoid abruptly stopping any psoriasis treatment without speaking with your doctor first – a transition to another drug may require an overlap period of using both treatments to avoid a possible flare or pustular eruption
- Avoid those drugs which are know to flare pustular psoriasis such as lithium, beta-blockers and others.
- Avoid irritating treatments such as coal tar medications when treating a severe, whole body psoriasis such as exfoliative erythroderma.

What is Psoriasis?

Further Reading:

What Causes Psoriasis? The most common question I get when I see a patient with psoriasis is "what caused it?" or "how did I get this?" The answer is complicated, but I've distilled it into the simple comment that "there is a genetic predisposition and usually a trigger factor that activates the disease". I think that's about as simplified an explanation as

you can get. A group of researchers in China compared 178 patients with psoriasis to 178 control patients with normal skin. What they found was that having the genetic HLA markers called HLA-Cw6 and HLA-B27 increased the risk of developing psoriasis by 2 to 10-fold. They also found that the risk of psoriasis was increased by environmental factors such as *manual work, marriage, stressful life events, obesity, family history of psoriasis and smoking.* So although you can't choose your parents, you can try to live a less stressful life, maintain normal body weight and don't start, or quit smoking. *I have no comment on the part about marriage!*

Newly Discovered Cells may Play a Role in Psoriasis Our skin has a complicated immune system which appears to be over-stimulated and overactive in psoriasis. Normally, cells called dendritic cells in the skin respond to infectious organisms by releasing cytokines which rev up the immune response to prepare for an attack. In psoriatic skin however there appears to be an additional population of very active "inflammatory dendritic cells" which are whipping the skin's immune system into a frenzy.

What is Psoriasis?

Does Stress Cause Psoriasis? One question almost all my patients with any sort of rash ask is "did stress cause this?" The answer is not straightforward, but it appears that stress plays

a role in people that are genetically predisposed to conditions such as eczema or psoriasis. A recent study showed that in mice, stress (in the form of an *unpleasant noise*) caused immune cells to enter the skin where they could release chemicals to increase itch (and possibly cause problems such as psoriasis). Not surprising then is the finding that meditation can help some patients with psoriasis. I wonder if the "unpleasant noise" used to stress the poor mice sound something like this: *"meow, meow"*?

What Causes Psoriasis, Part Two Most patients with psoriasis wonder what causes it, and at the fundamental level, it always goes back to genetics (although environmental factors seem to contribute as triggers). A new study involving some seven research institutes on both sides of the Atlantic have found some very interesting genetic links to psoriasis and psoriatic arthritis. They found the genes responsible for the link between psoriasis and elevated levels of inflammatory molecules called interleukins 12 and 23 and they also found genes which tie psoriasis and psoriatic arthritis to other autoimmune diseases. Previous genetic work with psoriasis has shown certain genetic markers to be more common in this disease, but the overall picture of how psoriasis is inherited remains enigmatic. *What causes psoriasis* is a puzzle we are still trying to put together.

It's in the Genes! A study looking at twins found that *skin psoriasis* was more likely to be shared among them than *psoriatic arthritis*. Another looked at a gene mutation which appears to account for 1.7% of psoriasis cases. It should be noted from this that psoriasis likely has many causes and many genes which affect it. Genes that are linked to psoriasis are termed *psoriasis susceptibility genes*.

Smoking Stongly Linked to Psoriasis A just published study looking at smoking and psoriasis concludes that both current and prior smoking increases the risk of psoriasis significantly. The risk of psoriasis was 37% higher among past smokers and 78% higher among current smokers than non-smokers. Your parents may have contributed more than their DNA to your psoriasis: exposure to passive smoke during pregnancy or childhood was associated with an increased risk of psoriasis. The risk of psoriasis among former smokers decreases very slowly and reaches that of non-smokers after nearly 20 years.

 Smoking is one of many lifestyle factors than can influence the severity of psoriasis.

Another Link in The Psoriasis Genetic Puzzle Found I like reading about genetic discoveries involving psoriasis because such information may in the long run lead to new and better treatments. Recently, scientists at the University of Nottingham in Britain looked at a particular gene know to cause inflammation in the skin called beta-defensin. They hypothesized that since this gene can trigger skin inflammation, psoriasis patients may be carrying extra copies of this gene. Studiying two different groups of patients, one in Germany and one in Netherlands, they confirmed their suspicions: *Psoriasis sufferers had significantly more copies of this inflammation-causing gene than other people*

Sunlight and Psoriasis: Friend, Foe, or *Both*?
Sunlight has been used to treat various diseases including Psoriasis since antiquity. There is little doubt that the ultraviolet

What is Psoriasis?

rays of the sun will clear Psoriasis for many patients. Using natural sunlight, or *Heliotherapy* to treat Psoriasis is not only effective, but essentially free assuming no lost work hours are involved. Many of my own patients experience a significant

clearing of their Psoriasis after moving to sunny Orlando from a more northern state.

Heliotherapy is easy when you have a private place to sun bathe and no worries about missing work at noontime. But what about apartment-dwellers whose only place to lay in the sun is at a shared pool or yard? More often than not I find that patients with moderate to severe Psoriasis would rather pass on Heliotherapy than to let their neighbors see the same rashy skin they otherwise take great care to hide or cover up.

Finding time, finding a place, and overcoming embarassment are just the up-front intangible costs of heliotherapy. Helio-therapy has late costs too, an "end load" if you will that should not be taken lightly: a signficantly increased risk of skin cancers and pre-cancers. This doesn't rule out heliotherapy as a useful tool, but it should be likened to other Psoriasis treatments all of which have their own risks, benefits, alternatives.

Psoriasis Impact Extends Beyond the Patients Themselves
A recent survey in Ireland noted that half the population has a family member or friend affected by Psoriasis, a surprisingly high number considering the often quoted statistic of a 2% prevalence for this disease. More than half those surveyed who were aware of Psoriasis felt it was difficult to live with. Although diet has been shown to play a very minimal role in Psoriasis, 50% thought that certain foods affected it.

What is Psoriasis?

Answering the Biggest Question of all: What Causes Psoriasis?

Researchers at the University of Texas M.D. Anderson Cancer Center have described how an excess amount of a natural

compound in the body may lead to psoriasis. The compound, LL37 or CAMP is released in a natural response to tissue injury

or infection and helps to stimulate a beneficial inflammatory response. In psoriasis it seems that there is too much of a good thing - LL37 continues to be produced in excess long after it is needed. The resulting chronic inflammation then leads to the inflamed skin lesions seen in psoriasis as well as several other autoimmune diseases.

Stories like this are exciting not just because they bring us closer to a full understanding of the nature of psoriasis, but because they hint at possible areas for drug development and

 treatment. Imagine an injection designed to bind excess LL37 and you'll immediately realize the potential of this research

Of course any practical application of this new data is many years away, but like I always tell my patients with psoriasis, there are new treatments for this disease being released every year. There is always hope for a better treatment and eventually, a cure.

Until then, LL37 appears to represent one more factor in the puzzling equation that explains the thickened, reddened and scaly skin plaques seen in psoriasis.

What is Psoriasis?

Section 2

Can Psoriasis be Prevented?
The short answer is yes and no. Like many diseases, psoriasis is influenced by both genetics *and* the environment.

The exact role these factors play is still a developing story, however we already have quite a bit of insight into how each can affect the course of psoriasis. Our genes are inherited from our parents, and certain genes may predispose us to develop psoriasis at some point in our lives.

For example, if a parent has psoriasis and one child develops the condition before age 15, siblings have a 50% chance of developing psoriasis, too. Identical twins have a 67% risk of sharing the disease. Certain HLA types can increase the risk of developing psoriasis by up to 6 times. Race can also be a predisposing genetic factor; those with fair-skin have a higher likelihood of developing the disease than darker-skinned individuals.

While you cannot change your genes, you can alter your environment and make choices that influence your risk of a psoriasis breakout.

Related Conditions
Managing related conditions may help you also fend off psoriasis. Stress, anxiety, depression and related emotional disorders can trigger psoriasis. In addition, psoriasis has been known to appear after an upper-respiratory tract infection, such strep throat or sinusitis. Psoriasis tends to be particularly severe in those with HIV/AIDS. Treating conditions such as these may also help keep psoriasis in check.

What is Psoriasis?

Medications

Certain medications can trigger or worsen psoriasis. These include:

- beta blockers and ACE inhibitors, used to treat high blood pressure
- the mood disorder drug lithium
- antimalarials related to hydroxychloroquine (which, today, are more likely to be prescribed for arthritis or lupus)

If it's an option for you, switching drugs or reducing your dose may help reduce risk of a psoriasis breakout.

Lifestyle

Of particular importance are those risk factors for which you have the most control over: physical environment, obesity, diet, alcohol consumption, and cigarette smoking.

Cold, dry air tends to worsen psoriasis, while a warm and humid climate is typically helpful, especially when natural sunlight can reach the skin. Although many reports have positioned obesity as a risk factor for psoriasis, one study demonstrated that obesity appears to be a *result of* psoriasis. A fruit and vegetable-rich "healthy" diet may be somewhat protective. Alcohol consumption increases the risk of developing and the severity of psoriasis to a small degree. Cigarette smoking worsens psoriasis with a demonstrable dose-response relationship implying a causal effect. Nevertheless, it is not entirely clear if alcohol and smoking are increased due to the stress of psoriasis or being a significant cause of the disease.

What is Psoriasis?

What You Can Do

You can't choose your parents (or your genes), but you *can* take measures to minimize the risks of psoriasis if you are genetically predisposed it. Remember to:

- Treat conditions associated the psoriasis breakouts early and thoroughly.
- Avoid medications known to flare psoriasis whenever possible.
- Maintain a normal body weight.
- Eat a diet rich in fresh fruits and vegetables.
- Eliminate or minimize smoking and alcohol.
- Keep skin moist with a humidifier and moisturizer.
- Plan moderate exposure to natural sunlight, without burning (take a walk outside on your lunch break, for example).

Which Medicines can Worsen Psoriasis?

Answer:

Some drugs can worsen psoriasis and should be avoided in those who have this disease. Several drugs or classes of drugs have been shown to worsen psoriasis. The major players in this phenomenon are:

Beta Blockers, such as *propranolol*. Used to treat high blood pressure patients and those who've experienced a heart attack, these drugs can worsen psoriasis within several weeks of starting the drug.

Lithium, used to treat bipolar disorders, can worsen psoriasis and even trigger psoriasis in people previously undiagnosed, sometimes as long as 15 months after starting the drug.

Antimalarials are drugs such as *hydroxychloroquine*, and they are typically used for the treatment of lupus or arthritis. Worsening of psoriasis has been reported with their use as early as 5 weeks into treatment.

Interferons, such as those used to treat hepatitis C, can aggravate existing or trigger new cases of psoriasis – and the condition may not improve after stopping the drug.

Other drugs that may worsen psoriasis include calcium channel blockers and angiotensin converting enzyme (ACE) inhibitors (for high blood pressure), the antifungal *terbenefine*, the smoking-cessation pill *bupropion* as well as SSRI-class antidepressants like *Prozac*

Avoid Skin Trauma to Minimize Psoriasis

Psoriasis adds Insult to Injury

One of the key features of psoriasis in many patients is a predilection for sites prone to chronic low-grade trauma such as elbows and knees. Certainly more direct trauma such as a cut or wound can *Koebnerize* or turn into psoriasis. For this reason, trauma to the skin needs to be avoided or minimized in psoriasis.

The Koebner phenomenon (Koebnerization, isomorphic response) occurs when a new area of psoriasis develops in injured skin. For example, after a surgery, psoriasis may develop around the surgical scar. This phenomenon may also help explain why psoriasis tends to occur on areas of constant low-intensity trauma such as elbows and knees. Koebnerization can occur after non-traumatic skin injury such as a sunburn, or an allergic reaction to a medication. In patients who suffer from dandruff or seborrheic dermatitis of

What is Psoriasis?

the face and scalp, psoriasis can superimpose itself due to irritation and scratching and a crossover or combination dermatitis known as "sebopsoriasis" develops. Koebnerization is not specific to psoriasis.

Recently a patient of mine who was quite stable and completely clear of psoriasis while under treatment with Efalizumab came to the office with a severe outbreak of psoriasis on the fingers. After a bit a questioning, the reason became clear. He had installed a fence a few days earlier and sustained repeated trauma to his fingers in the process. Over the next month or so, his regular treatment cleared the psoriasis but he'll be much more careful next time!

Koebnerization can occur after indirect or even non-physical trauma as well. I've seen sunburns and allergic drug reactions turn into psoriasis. It's heartbreaking to see when someone who was trying to clear their psoriasis with sunlight ends up even worse due to a sunburn induced whole-body flare up.

Baby your skin to keep it calm. Minimize all sorts of trauma and you'll be one step closer to preventing outbreaks of psoriasis.

Psoriasis Flare

A Severe and Sudden Worsening of Psoriasis

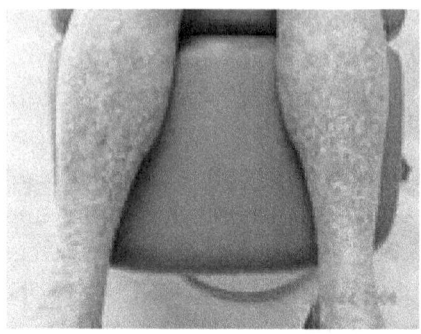

Rapidly Worsening Psoriasis © *New Paradigm Dermatology, PL*

One of the more distressing features of psoriasis is the occasional sudden and severe worsening of symptoms, often without any obvious cause. A closer look however may yield several clues as to possible inciting factors. Treatment of flares can be challenging, and in worst cases, may require a brief hospitalization. Most psoriasis flares however can be handled with systemic medications in the setting of the doctor's office.

Causes of Flares

Several triggering factors have been identified as contributing to worsening psoriasis:

- External Factors: Nearly any injury to the skin can result in the development or worsening of psoriasis including sunburn, other rashes like allergic reaction to drugs, surgery, cuts or scratches, and viral rashes. The worsening of psoriasis after injury is known as the Koebner phenomenon.

What is Psoriasis?

- Infections: Most notoriously, streptococcal infections such as strep throat can trigger the disease, especially an outbreak of guttate psoriasis. HIV infection is another condition known to aggravate psoriasis.
- Psychological Stress: Job loss, divorice, death or other major emotional upsets have been known to flare psoriasis weeks or months after the stressful event.
- Medications: Many medications are known to trigger psoriasis and should be avoided in patients with the disease.

Treating Psoriasis Flares

At one time, hospitalization for psoriasis flares was common. Due to changes in insurance reimbursement (Medicare only allows so many days of hospitalization for a skin condition) and more powerful and faster acting drugs, most flares are treated in the outpatient setting.

Drugs commonly used for severe flares include cyclosporine, Remicade (infliximab), and for pustular flares, Soriatane (acetretin). When psoriasis flares, don't delay – seek treatment urgently with a qualified dermatologist.

Further Reading:

Beta Blockers Exonerated? Looking at the colossal U.K.-based General Practice Research Database, researchers out of Geneva and Boston concluded that beta blocker medications did not increase the risk of first-time psoriasis diagnosis. I'm not entirely convinced however – I've seen pustular psoriasis develop in previously undiagnosed patients when put on beta blockers and plaque type psoriasis get worse or more difficult to manage in conjunction with beta blockers. Perhaps then

---

What is Psoriasis?

beta blockers don't cause psoriasis but may tend to make it worse? That's another study!

Section 3

Mimics of Psoriasis

These Things Aren't Psoriasis but Often Look Like it

Many rashes can cause skin changes just like psoriasis. With careful inspection, it should be possible to differentiate these psoriasis posers from the real thing. Psoriasis is most likely to be confused with another rash based on the location of the rash. For example many things can cause a red scaly rash in the groin area other than psoriasis.

Scalp Rashes That Aren't Psoriasis

Scaly red rashes on the scalp can be caused by seborrheic dermatitis, also known as *dandruff*. The difference is that psoriasis of the scalp often has significant thickening of the skin and thick adherent scales. Seborrheic dermatitis usually just has some pinkness of the skin of the scalp with much finer scales. Seborrheic dermatitis often involves the eyebrows and the sides of the nostrils as well, so sometimes involvement of these areas will help to separate this disease from psoriasis.

Fungal infections of the scalp are not so rare in children and so a child with a scaly scalp may have fungus, psoriasis or seborrheic dermatitis. Hairs can be plucked and examined under a microscope to help confirm a diagnosis of fungus.

Flexural Area Rashes that Aren't Psoriasis

In the creases of the armpits and groin area, as well as under breasts, the increased moisture present tends to macerate scales creating a pasty white substance. Redness and maceration can be seen with both psoriasis or *candidiasis* (common yeast infection). A dryer red rash with scales around the edges

What is Psoriasis?

is typical of *tinea cruris* or "Jock Itch". A darker discolored patch in this area without scaliness may be *erythrasma*, a minor bacterial infection. Your dermatologist can examine skin scales or debris under a microscope or use an ultraviolet light called a *Wood's Light* to help differentiate these rashes from psoriasis.

Hand and Foot Rashes that Aren't Psoriasis
Hand and foot rashes may be the most difficult to differentiate from true psoriasis. Eczema, fungal infections, allergic reactions and irritation from chemicals can all cause changes which may be confused with psoriasis. Most of these rashes cause thickening, redness and scales on the backs of the hands or feet but may cause a blistering rash on the palms and soles. Nail changes can occur in fungus or severe eczema involving the cuticle areas. Skin biopsies from hand and foot rashes can be confusing and often show mixed features of both psoriasis *and* eczema in the same specimen. Differentiating hand and foot rashes from psoriasis requires significant skill and usually necessitates examination of other body parts, ie: scalp, elbows, knees, to look for clues.

Psoriasis vs. Eczema

Similar, but Different
Both psoriasis and eczema are chronic skin diseases that cause red, scaly skin rashes. Though they are quite similar, the range of symptoms for each is usually different enough for your doctor to tell them apart without doing a skin biopsy or other diagnostic testing.

Psoriasis lesions are typically thick, red, and scaly (dry). Although eczema lesions may be similar if they are chronic, they also can appear as moist and oozing areas. Both tend to affect the hands, feet, and nape of the neck. When the problem is in these areas, it can be difficult for even a doctor to distinguish one condition from another. But, there are some telltale signs: Psoriasis likes to involve the back of the elbows and front of the knees (extensor surfaces), while eczema favors the inside of the arms and the back of the knees (flexor surfaces). Both rashes appear frequently on the scalp, while chronic eczema is found on the ankles more often than psoriasis.

Hands and feet are the most difficult areas to tell psoriasis and eczema apart. For one thing, fungus may be along for the ride as well. Even a biopsy of hand and foot rashes may show confusing overlap, causing pathologists to "hedge" a bit and give a non-specific reading or report. One small clue to psoriasis of the hands is that nails will show pitting. Nail changes also occur in eczema and fungus cases, but pitting – especially in a nail where *the cuticle is not involved with any rashes* – is fairly uncommon. Fortunately, both psoriasis and eczema of the hands and feet will respond to topical steroid creams, so treatment is usually not hindered by this diagnostic confusion.

Some treatments work for both psoriasis and eczema, though others are quite specific. It's important to see a dermatologist so that you rash can be assessed and you can get the most effective treatment.

Reiter Syndrome

A Trio of Seemingly Unrelated Symptoms
Reiter syndrome, also known as reactive arthritis with conjunctivitis / urethritis / diarrhea, is a rare disease with psoriasis-like symptoms which often occurs after a bacterial infection. The syndrome often follows an infectious urethritis (infection of the tube that carries urine from the bladder to

the genital area) or infectious diarrhea. It is more common in patients who have the genetic marker called HLA-B27 (as is psoriasis). Symptoms include inflammation of the eyes, arthritis and a thick scaly foot rash which mimics psoriasis called *keratoderma blenorrhagicum*. Initial treatments include conservative measures such as range-of-motion exercises and joint injections of anti-inflammatory steroid medications. Fore more severe cases, methotrexate, infliximab, acetretin and cyclosporine may be used.

The disease is named after Hans Reiter, who unfortunately was also a Nazi war criminal involved in involuntary sterilization and concentration camp experiments involving typhus. For this reason the much more cumbersome *reactive arthritis with conjunctivitis/urethritis/diarrhea* moniker is sometimes preferred.

Take-Home Message
If your stubborn foot psoriasis is accompanied by eye inflammation and arthritis and was preceded by a bacterial infection, you may wish to ask your doctor about the possibility of Reiter syndrome.

Cutanteous T-Cell Lymphoma or CTCL

A skin cancer which can mimic psoriasis

Looks Like Psoriasis, but it's not
Cutaneous T-Cell Lymphoma, or CTCL for short, often appears as persistent scaly red patches which look quite similar to psoriasis. To make diagnosis more confusing, a skin biopsy of a lesion of CTCL may not show the disease until a patient has had the condition *for up to 7 years*. Another name for the most common type of CTCL is *mycosis fungoides* but this name

What is Psoriasis?

is slowly fading from use since it sounds like it pertains to a fungal infection and not a malignancy.

How it Differs from Psoriasis

In the long run, lesions of CTCL often evolve from a flat or patch stage to a raised or plaque stage and finally to large lesions called tumor stage. Lymph nodes can be enlarged and malignant white blood cells called *Sezary cells* can be found in the bloodstream.

Treatment of CTCL

Early stages of CTCL often respond to the same types of treatments as psoriasis such as topical steroids or phototherapy. Later stages may need chemotherapy or a CTCL-specific retinoid drug called targretin.

Treatment of Advanced Cases of CTCL

Generally speaking, advanced cases of CTCL are more likely to be treated by an oncologist than a dermatologist. A form of phototherapy called *extracorporeal photopheresis* where blood is removed from the body and exposed to ultraviolet light can be used in advanced cases as well as total body electron beam therapy, a type of radiation therapy. Advanced cases of CTCL which do not respond to any of these therapies are treated with even newer medications. An interesting drug called Ontak is approved for use of CTCL. Ontak is made by fusing diphtheria toxin to the cytokine IL-2. When it binds to the IL-2 receptors present on CTCL cells, they die. Zolina is used for CTCL when other treatments have already failed. It alters the malignant cells' DNA metabolism. Both Ontak and Zolina have been associated with severe side effects.

What Should I do with This Information?

If you have a stubborn rash, which is somewhat atypical for psoriasis and it has not responded well to treatment, it may be worthwhile to consider a skin biopsy of a lesion to determine if features of CTCL or psoriasis are present. In many cases, the rash of CTCL may preceed a definitive biopsy diagnosis by several years, hence in some patients repeated serial skin biopsies over many years may be required to *confirm* a diagnosis of CTCL.

Pityriasis Rubra Pilaris

When It Looks Like Psoriasis, But It's Not

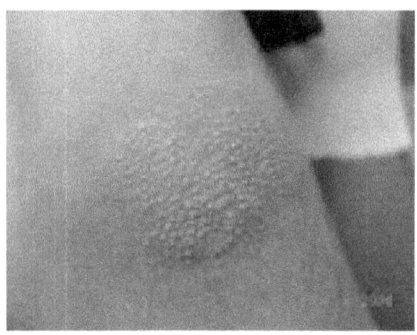

distinct, follicular keratotic papules in a red plaque ©*New Paradigm Dermatology, PL*

Pityriasis rubra pilaris (PRP), like psoriasis, is a skin disease caused by problems with keratinization – the scientific term for the normal growth and maturation of skin cells. Psoriasis and PRP rashes look so similar that sometimes a skin biopsy is needed to tell them apart.

What Causes PRP?

What is Psoriasis?

The exact cause is unknown and since PRP is much rarer than psoriasis, there has been less research done on the disease.

Similarities and Differences Between PRP and Psoriasis

Both diseases:

- can cause thickening, reddening and scaliness of the palms and soles
- can cause red skin plaques on other areas of the body
- can affect fingernails and toenails
- may lead to the Koebner response where an injury to the skin can produce the rash itself.

Differences: PRP causes the presence of *distinct follicular-based papules*. In other words, there are small hard plugs in every skin follicle, versus the more scaly appearance of psoriasis.

Treatment of PRP
PRP may get better just by doing simple things like using moisturizers or keratolytics. It can also be treated with phototherapy, methotrexate and retinoid drugs like Soriatane. In many cases, RPR goes away completely over time.

Further Reading

The Dandruff-Psoriasis Connection Both dandruff (seborrheic dermatitis) and psoriasis can cause redness, flaking and itching, but technically they remain different diseases. Clinically there are areas of overlap, for example when patients prone to both conditions have psoriasis-like rashes in the areas typically involved by seborrheic dermatitis (face, scalp, underarms and groin). Such combinations are often termed

---

What is Psoriasis?

"sebopsoriasis" since they share features of both diseases. A recent study out of Iran looked at the cause of dandruff (a yeast called Malassezia furfur) and found that psoriasis lesions

tended to be colonized with a form of Malassezia that encourages inflammation. Perhaps this then is the "missing like" between these to disorders?

Section 4

Overview of Psoriatic Arthritis

Psoriatic arthritis (PsA) is a condition that is associated with the skin condition psoriasis. It is an inflammatory type of arthritis that causes stiff joints, among other symptoms.

How Common is Psoriatic Arthritis?
About a third of patients with psoriasis have some degree of joint stiffness. A true inflammatory arthritis affects 6 to 10% of patients with moderate to severe psoriasis. There is some genetic overlap in the two diseases, but there are also some genetic markers that are more common in PsA than psoriasis.

What Triggers Psoriatic Arthritis?
It is not known exactly what causes PsA, but there are several theories: "deep" Koebner phenomenon, emotional stress, and bacterial infections have all been proposed as triggers. Like psoriatic skin, the joint space in psoriatic arthritis shows high levels of TNF-alpha. Biologic drugs that block TNF-alpha are extremely effective in treating PsA.

Risk Factors for Psoriatic Arthritis
Several factors have been correlated with PsA. It is more common in Caucasian people and those who have a relative with PsA. Although children can be afflicted with PsA, adults between the ages of 30 to 50 are at highest risk. Being HIV positive increases the likelihood of PsA.

What is Psoriasis?

The Patterns of Psoriatic Arthritis

Five distinct patterns of arthritis are seen in PsA, and once a particular pattern in established in any given patient, it is unlikely to change:

- **Symmetric Polyarthritis**
  This most common form of PsA can involve any joint, but it typically involves the knuckles near the hands, and is very similar to rheumatoid arthritis.
- **Asymmetric Oligoarticular Arthritis**
  Typically, five or fewer joints in fingers or toes are inflamed creating a distinct "sausage digit" type of swelling known as *dactylitis*.
- **Distal Interphalangeal Joint Arthritis**
  In this form, the joints further away from the knuckles are involved; psoriatic nail changes are seen in almost all cases.
- **Arthritis Mutilans**
  This severe form of arthritis fortunately represents only 1 to 2% of PsA. It is more common in early onset psoriasis and has the worst prognosis, or outcome.
- **Sacroiliitis and Spine Pain**
  X-ray findings of sacroiliitis (inflammation where the tailbone or sacrum meets the hipbone or ilium) help distinguish PSA from rheumatoid arthritis. X-ray findings similar to ankylosis spondylitis can also be seen, but lumbosacral stiffness and range of motion loss in PsA is not as severe.

Other Features of PsA

Sometimes, there are other symptoms with PsA such as fever, fatigue and loss of appetite. PsA symptoms usually appear after skin psoriasis is evident, but less frequently occur at the same time or even before psoriasis of the skin appears. When

What is Psoriasis?

PsA and psoriasis are occurding together, it is often difficult for a doctor to differentiate PsA from rheumatoid arthritis when blood test results are not conclusive (ie: rheumatoid factor or RF for rheumatoid arthritis is negative). Blood tests which may be altered in PsA include CBC, platelet counts, erythrocyte sedimentation rate, C-reactive Protein, and uric acid. In the near future, a new blood test for antibodies to something called "proteosomes" may be helpful in diagnosing PsA when and if it becomes commercially available.

Since there is no single specific confirmatory test for PsA, the diagnosis of this disease remains a clinical one which usually relies on the the overall findings as assessed by a rheumatologist.

Nail pitting is more common in psoriasis patients with PSA than without. Serious eye problems including iritis, conjunctivitis and anterior uveitis can be seen in a minority of patients with PSA.

Further Reading:

Psoriatic Arthritis Trigger Factors Psoriatic arthritis typically follows the development of skin psoriasis in those who get this condition. What is not currently known is what may trigger the development of psoriatic arthritis. A recent study surveyed 98 patients with recent onset of psoriatic arthritis and compared them to controls without the disease. Pre-disposing factors seen more commonly in patients with psoriatic arthritis vs. controls were: Rubella vaccination; Trauma; Oral ulcerations; Moving; and Bone fracture requiring hospital admission.

A very interesting hodge-podge of seemingly completely unrelated phenomena indeed!

What is Psoriasis?

Psoriatic arthritis: Cause and Effect Two new studies about psoriatic arthritis in the news this week. The first study looked at a high incidence of autoantibodies to proteosomes in psoriatic arthritis patients. Proteosomes are small intracellular structures involved in protein recycling, breaking down old proteins into amino acid building blocks so that they can be used to manufacture new proteins. The autoantibodies called *anti-20s* were even more elevated in systemic lupus erythematosus patients, so they were not specific for psoriatic arthritis, although they were relatively rare in rheumatoid arthritis patients and may help in differentiating these two diseases.

The other study showed a link between psoriatic arthritis and atherosclerosis. They looked at the thickness of the blood vessel walls in the carotid arteries and found that they were thicker in patients with psoriatic arthritis than in control patients. I think this one once again confirms that patients with psoriasis (or in this case, psoriatic arthritis) need to have very thorough physical exams and medical follow up with their primary care physicians to look for associated medical problems.

Anti-Oxidants Good for Psoriatic Arthritis?
A group of researchers in Rome noted that two compounds which measure protein oxidation are reduced in in the synovial (joint fluid) of patients with psoriatic arthritis. The same markers are inversely correlated to the levels of CRP, a marker for inflammation i.e. the more inflammation, the more protein oxidation and the less the levels of these two compounds are. Could it be that anti-oxidants may be helpful for patients with psoriatic arthritis?

Section 5

Psoriasis – More than Just Skin Deep

Psoriasis Heralds Increased Risk for Several Serious Diseases
I'll be honest with you. If you have psoriasis, what you doctor *doesn't know* might kill you. Strong words? Yes, but lately so much data is accumulating about psoriasis and general health that this topic is taking on great importance – much more so than when I trained as a dermatologist. Most doctors in practice today probably still look at psoriasis as simply a skin rash. We now know that psoriasis can be an indicator of many more serious underlying conditions. Both you and your doctor need to be aware of the risks associated with having psoriasis.

Case in point: Research on the United Kingdom's colossal General Practice Research Database (GPRD) – a bank of information on 9 million patients, more than 100,000 of whom have a diagnosis of psoriasis. Researchers looked for trends, and found some eye-opening information we had better pay close attention to.

Psoriasis and the Risk of Lymphoma
Psoriasis, like rheumatoid arthritis (RA), is an autoimmune condition that has been associated with an increased risk of lymphoma. There are several types of lymphoma, at least two of which are increased in patients with psoriasis by as much as 10-fold over patients without the skin condition.

Lymphoma is a cancer of white blood cells which typically leads to swollen lymph nodes. Many lymph nodes are superficial and can be palpated (felt) by your physician during a routine exam. If enlarged lymph nodes are felt, they can be further investigated.

Psoriasis and the Risk of Heart Attack

Moderate to severe psoriasis can pose as much as a 3-fold increase for the risk of a heart attack. Chronic inflammation, as is seen in psoriasis, is now believed to be a major player in the development of heart disease. Blood tests, such as C-reactive protein (CRP), are often done to screen for risk of heart attack and should be a routine part of your lab work if you have moderate to severe psoriasis. If you have other risk factors for heart disease, such as diabetes, high blood pressure, or obesity, make sure you and your doctor address these aggressively as well.

Severe Psoriasis and Increased Risk of Death

In the U.K. study, the risk of overall mortality (death) was increased in people with severe psoriasis by roughly 50%, with these patients experiencing about a 4-year shorter life span. Though worth noting, these figures are less troublesome than those from other research in Canada. In this study, life expectancy was decreased by 10 years over the Canadian average; for those who developed psoriasis before age 25, life expectancy was decreased by *25 to 30 years*. A truly startling statistic.

What Else Can Psoriasis Patients Do?

In addition to the above, the Canadian study found that diabetes and genitourinary (reproductive and urinary) diseases were more common in psoriasis patients. The lead researcher suggested that psoriasis patients get regular blood pressure, blood sugar, and lipid tests, as well as electrocardiograms.

What is Psoriasis?

Let Your Physician Know
The information presented here is relatively new. Do yourself a favor – let your physician know that you are concerned. While the screenings mentioned here may be a part of your routine physical, it is certainly a good idea to discuss the association of psoriasis and these other conditions with your doctor.

Psoriasis, Obesity and Heart Disease

Which Comes First and What Does it Matter?

Background
Psoriasis is a condition of chronic inflammation marked by increased levels of TNF-alpha. It has also been associated with obesity with at least one study concluding that *obesity is a result rather than a cause* of psoriasis. Less well known is the link between TNF-alpha and obesity.

TNF-alpha:Obesity Connection
It seems that TNF-alpha makes obese rodents put on more weight. Current thought is that TNF-alpha may play a key role in the control of body mass.

TNF-alpha, Psoriasis and Myocardial Infarction
TNF-alpha also causes changes in the body that increase the risk of myocardial infarction. It's not surprising then that psoriasis itself has been shown to increase a person's risk of myocardial infarction.

Should This Affect the Way We Treat Psoriasis?
The relationship between chronic inflammation and overweight in psoriasis is the subject of a new clinical trial at Harvard. Overweight psoriasis patients will be studied with

medications that reduce the levels of TNF-alpha in the body. The results should be interesting at many levels.

I Have Psoriasis. Am I At Risk For Other Conditions?

Question: I Have Psoriasis. Am I At Risk For Other Conditions?
People with psoriasis, especially severe psoriasis, may be at risk for several other serious conditions, such as cardiovascular disease, hypertension, obesity, diabetes, heart attack, depression and early death. How do you screen for and reduce the risk of these conditions?

Answer:
In recent years more attention has been paid to the association between moderate to severe psoriasis and seemingly unrelated conditions like heart disease and cancer. What we are learning is that if you have moderate to severe psoriasis, you may in fact be at a somewhat higher risk of developing other medical problems too. If you have psoriasis, you may want to check out screening guidelines through the American Heart Association and American Cancer Society. Psoriasis itself may be an independent risk factor for many other conditions. Make sure your primary care physician is aware of this increased risk so that appropriate monitoring can be scheduled.

Psoriasis and Cardiovascular Disease
Psoriasis patients are at increased risk for cardiovascular disease and heart attack, independent of other risk factors such as obesity and smoking. In addition, many psoriatics are overweight and smoke, compounding the risk. Here are the American Heart Association recommendations for cardiovascular disease risk factor screening:

- blood pressure; body mass index (BMI); waist circumference and pulse: *monitored at least every two years.* BP should be below 120/80 mm HG; BMI <25 and waist circumference less than 35 in. for women and < 40 in. for men.
- fasting cholesterol panel and blood glucose: *monitored at least every 5 years, or every 2 years if other risk factors are present such as family history, diabetes, or smoking.* Total cholesterol should be less than 200, HDL great than or equal to 50, LDL <100 and blood glucose <100.
- moderate to intense physical activity at least 30 minutes most days of the week and healthy eating.

Psoriasis and Malignancy

Cancers noted with increased frequency in psoriasis include Hodgkin's lymphoma, cutaneous T-cell lymphoma (CTCL), and cutaneous squamous cell carcinoma (SCC). Various other cancers of internal organs may be noted with increased frequency in patients with psoriasis, however the other causes of cancer such as smoking, alcohol and the use of cancer-causing psoriasis treatments make measuring the risk of these cancers difficult. Here are the American Cancer Society screening recommendations:

- General Clinical Exam: Recommended for those 20 years and older, looking for cancer of the thyroid, oral cavity, skin, lymph nodes, testes, and or ovaries
- Breast Cancer: Ages 20-39: breast exam every three years; Ages 40 and older: annual breast exam and annual mammogram.
- Colon and Rectal cancer: For age 50 and over: fecal occult blood test or immunochemical test annually, flexible sigmoidoscopy every 5 years, double-contrast

   barium enema every 5 years, colonoscopy every 10 years
- Prostate cancer: Over age 50, PSA blood test and digital rectal exam annually.

Other Recommendations

Reducing other known risk factors for cancer and heart disease are probably more important for those with psoriasis than without. Smoking cessation, reducing alcohol intake and monitoring for depression are all useful adjuncts to the above screening guidelines

---

Further Reading:

Risks of Depression in Psoriasis Patients with psoriasis are up to 2.7 times more likely to be diagnosed with depression compared to patients without psoriasis. Using reports from 150 million dermatology visits logged into the National Ambulatory Medical Care Survey and the National Hospital Ambulatory Care Survey, researchers found 4.7 million visits for psoriasis. They then compared this figure to the number of patients diagnosed with depression.

They found that the risk of depression was 4.5 times more likely in younger patients (age 40 and under) with psoriasis. The risk was also elevated, but less so, in those over age 40 (1.8 times more likely). They attributed this difference to the significant effects of psoriasis on socializing, finding a partner and establishing a career in younger persons suffering from this disease. The degree of depression has also been correlated with the degree of itch in some patients.

What is Psoriasis?

Psoriasis and the Risk of Diabetes An article in the British Journal of Dermatology looked at the rate of new-onset diabetes developing in patients with psoriasis. They took their data from the UK –based *General Practice Research Database*. The Risk of developing diabetes was higher in those patients with psoriasis. The severity of the psoriasis was what related to the risk of diabetes, not the BMI (body mass index) which would have related it to obesity instead (another common finding in diabetes). Psoriasis is being looked at more and more as a marker or risk factor for many other serious conditions.

More on Psoriasis and Heart Disease The current issue of the American Journal of Cardiology contains a consensus document by dermatologists and cardiologists regarding the increased risk of cardiovascular disease in patients with psoriasis. The relationship between heart disease and psoriasis has been noted since 1961. Large epidemiological studies done since then have added support to the idea that psoriasis patients are indeed at risk for heart disease. The consensus statement recommends that two groups of psoriasis patients be evaluated for vascular disease: those with moderate to severe psoriasis; and those with mild psoriasis plus a recognized risk factor for vascular disease such as abdominal obesity or hypertension.

Psoriasis, Homocysteine and Heart Disease A really interesting study from Turkey looked at serum homocysteine levels in patients with psoriasis. Elevated homocysteine levels are a recognized risk factor for heart disease. More recently, psoriasis itself has been proposed as an independent risk factor for heart disease. Two interesting finding from the study should be mentioned. Firstly, overall homocysteine levels did not differ significantly between psoriasis patients and controls. Second, and of possible clinical importance to patients is that homocysteine levels *did* correlate with the *severity* of psoriasis. One conclusion that could possibly be raised by such data is that reducing the severity of psoriasis may in fact reduce the severity of heart disease. Although this has not been studied in and of itself, it may change the risk/benefit profiles of many treatments. The side effects of some psoriasis treatments may be more acceptable if in fact heart disease risk is also being mitigated.

Obesity and Psoriasis Symptoms In a study looking at siblings with and without psoriasis, researchers found that psoriasis was more common in an obese sibling, at least among women. For both men and women however, an increased BMI (body mass index) was associated with worsening psoriasis. Just another peek at the association between obesity and psoriasis.

Obesity and Psoriasis Treatment We know that obesity is associated with psoriasis. Perhaps obesity increases the risk of psoriasis, or perhaps the genetic and environmental factors that cause psoriasis increase the risk of obesity. In any case, a recent study looked at the benefits of losing weight on the effectiveness of cyclosprorine on psoriasis. Twice as many patients that lost 7% of their body weight on a low calorie diet achieved PASI 75 improvement vs. the control group. I'd suspect that the effect of weight loss on psoriasis treatment is probably not limited to cyclosporine.

Psoriasis Patients at Increased Risk for Diabetes According to data compiled from the United Kingdom's General Practice Research Database (GPRD), patients with psoriasis are more likely to develop diabetes. The overall risk for developing diabetes was 31% higher in psoriasis patients but the risk of diabetes developing increased the longer the patient has had

What is Psoriasis?

psoriasis. Severe psoriasis requiring more than 2 systemic prescriptions per year increased the risk of diabetes by 77%.

Obesity Increases Psoriasis Risk A relatively new thought in genetic medicine is that genes can be switched on and off depending upon "environmental conditions" in other words, lifestyle. Here we have a study that links obesity with an increased risk of psoriasis, specifically related to one psoriasis-promoting gene. Obesity, like smoking and alcohol is a lifestyle issue which seems to have a significant effect on the severity and response to treatment of psoriasis.

Psoriasis and Weight Gain: Cause or Effect?
Obesity has been linked to psoriasis, but there is still some confusion as to whether or not obesity *causes* psoriasis, or (less pondered, but no less likely) obesity is caused by psoriasis. Some studies published in Obesity Surgery in 2004 and 2006 looked at weight gain and psoriasis. They referenced the 78,000+ subject Nurses' Health Study II which has been a tremendous source of epidemiology and lifestyle health data. There was a strong correlation between body-mass index (BMI, a measure of possible obesity) and incidence of psoriasis with a nearly three times greater risk of psoriasis in those with higher BMIs. There have also been case reports of patient's psoriasis clearing up after tremendous weight loss, i.e. after gastric bypass surgery

One explaination may involve the pro-inflammatory role that body fat, especially intra-abdominal fat plays and the secretion of substances that promote psoriasis for example, TNF-alpha. It should be noted that blocking TNF-alpha is a the mechanism by which many biologic medicines for psoriasis work. If indeed, obesity leads to psoriasis, it provides another target for lifestyle alteration in the fight against this disease.

What is Psoriasis?

Severe Psoriasis Linked to Higher Risk for Stroke Looking at the UK General Practice Research Database, a University of Pennsylvania researcher noted a slightly increased risk for stroke among those with severe psoriasis. The numbers amounted to one additional stroker per 530 patients per year, not a large number but about a 6% increased risk vs. those without psoriasis. The increased risk was not associated with any particular treatment used. The reason for the association is unknown, but may lie in the common feature of psoriasis, acute myocardial infarction and stroke which is excess inflammation.

Pulmonary Hypertension More Common in Psoriasis Pulmonary hypertension is a slowly progressive process which often goes undiagnosed until late in the course of the disease. A new study links psoriasis with pulmonary hypertension. Pulmonary hypertension was found in about a third of psoriasis patients, and none of the control patients. Just another general health issue to be looked for in patients with psoriasis.

More than Skin Deep, Revisited This month's *Journal of Drugs in Dermatology* has a study looking at data collected for the National Health and Wellness Survey (40,000 patients including 1127 psoriasis patients). Several conditions were more likely in those with psoriasis than controls including: diabetes, hypertension, hypercholesterolemia, congestive heart failure, anxiety, arthritis, chronic obstructive pulmonary disease, depression, gastroesophageal reflux, and insomnia. Here's the usual disclaimer again: if you have moderate to severe psoriasis, you need a primary care physician who is really on top of all the increased risks you may face as a patient with this disease. For more on general health and psoriasis, look here.

What is Psoriasis?

More on Celiac disease and Psoriasis A possible link between psoriasis and celiac disease has already been established – antibodies to gliadin a component of wheat and other grasses is present in both diseases. A new study published in the Journal of the European Academy of Dermatology and Venereology confirmed the link and found that severity of psoriasis correlated with the level of anti-gliadin antibodies meaning the antibodies may play a role in the development of this disease.

Itch, Depression and Psoriasis A German psoriasis study found a link between pruritus (itch) and depression in psoriasis. The study didn't touch on mechanism, although I find it interesting that inflammatory markers in the blood such as IL-6 can be increased in depression as well as psoriasis. Itch and pain follow the same nerves and utilize the same parts of the brain as well and the link between chronic pain and depression is already known. Listening to music, which seems to help *chronic pain and depression* could also help the *itch and depression* of psoriasis.

Diabetes twice as common in Psoriasis A pre-publication release of a study in the Journal of the European Academy of Dermatology and Venereology looked at the incidence of diabetes in 16,000 plus psoriasis patients and around 75,000 controls. The study was done in Israel. In those patients over age 35, the proportion of diabetics with psoriasis was significantly higher. Patients with psoriasis had a 58% increased risk of diabetes. Some 13.8% of psoriasis had diabetes while only 5.4% of the controls had diabetes. If you have psoriasis, keep a close eye on your weight and make sure to have your fasting blood glucose checked at your annual physical.

What is Psoriasis?

Beneficial Side Effects of a Diabetes Med An article in the Journal of the American Academy of Dermatology looked at the relationship between the use of thiazolidinedione drugs for diabetes (such as actos) and psoriasis. Looking at the massive UK General Practice Research Database they found a negative correlation between the use of these drugs and initial diagnosis of psoriasis – in other words *they seem to protect against psoriasis.* This is somewhat reminiscent of the beneficial side effect of simvastatin on psoriasis. While there is no clear-cut recommendation on the use of diabetes and cholesterol drugs in psoriasis, those psoriasis patients with diabetes or high lipids may want to make note of the medications out there which may offer dual benefits for them.

The "Heartbreak" of Psoriasis In the March 2008 *Journal of the American Academy of Dermatology* is a thorough review called "Psoriasis: The Heart of the Matter" which looks at increased risk of heart disease in association with psoriasis. The article reviewed several important findings:

-the risk of atherosclerotic heart disease has been linked to low grade inflammation as indicated by blood markers such as TNF-a (which happens to be greatly increased in psoriasis).

-risk factors for heart disease such as smoking, obesity, diabetes, hypertension and elevated lipids are all associated with severe psoriasis as well

-and then there is the recent study (mentioned above) which shows that severe psoriasis is a risk factor for coronary artery disease, independent of these several shared risk factors, ie: smoking, obesity, etc.

What is Psoriasis?

With the evidence piled high regarding heart disease and diabetes, I'd like to once again urge readers with severe psoriasis to check in with their primary care doctors to make sure that they have been thoroughly assessed for coronary artery disease. And remember, psoriasis is much more than *skin deep*.

Treatment for Diabetes Reduces Psoriasis Risk A new study in the Journal of the American Academy of Dermatology found that patients treated with certain anti-diabetic medications were at reduced risk of developing psoriasis. They also found that smoking and obesity were risk factors for developing psoriasis, something we've noted before in this blog.

Smoking and overweight are just two lifestyle issues associated with psoriasis.

Is Psoriasis More Dangerous than Hypertension? Archives of Dermatology has an article re-iterrating that indeed severe psoriasis does pose a risk to the general health of patients and may decrease life expectancy by several years (more so than hypertension). The increased overall inflammation produced by psoriasis may be damaging the cardiovascular system in patients with severe disease. Notably, many drugs for psoriasis such as Enbrel are designed to reduce inflammation. Perhaps such drugs provide benefits beyond just treating the skin? Time will tell.

A Beneficial Side-Effect: Simvastatin Helps Clear Psoriasis In a preliminary study published in *Journal of the American Academy of Dermatology*, the cholesterol-lowering drug Simvastatin (brand name Zocor®) was able to *decrease* the severity of psoriasis. Usually we hear about how patients with Psoriasis have to avoid certain drugs which may flare their skin disease. It's a pleasant surprise to hear the opposite for a change. Seven patients with Psoriasis were treated with Simvastatin 40mg daily for 8 weeks. There was a statistically significant reduction in the severity of their skin disease (average improvement 47%). One patient dropped out of the study due to headaches. Two patients achieved a 75% improvement. These values are impressive, as good as some drugs we currently use to treat Psoriasis. Such a small study needs to be reinforced with additional numbers before we can begin to tout simvastatin or any of the related statin drugs as psoriasis treatments. But if you are going to be starting a cholesterol-lower drug anyway and are already suffering from Psoriasis, you may wish to let your doctor know about the *potential* dual benefits of this drug for you.

The Heavy Psychological Burden of Psoriasis and the Benefits of Intervention Psoriasis-specific group psychological intervention can be a powerful tool not just in learning to deal with the emotional burdens of the disease, but in treating the disease itself. It seems that talking about your Psoriasis with others similarly afflicted can actually help to clear your skin more quickly and effectively. Psoriasis patients like others with significant skin diseases tend to suffer tremendous amounts of stress regarding their skin. While appearance plays a part in this, it is actually issues regarding perceived control and the demands of the condition that fuels this stress. The good news is that there is evidence that psychological intervention can provide many benefits including a reduction in unhelpful beliefs about the condition, as well as anxiety, depression and stress. Not just the mind, but the body improves: physician-rated clinic severity improved and three times more people achieved 75% clearing of their skin compared to patients not receiving adjunctive psychological treatment.

Section 6

Coal Tar Products for Psoriasis

Ancient Remedy – New Worries?

Long before steroids, there was coal tar. In fact, coal tar has been used in the treatment of skin diseases for over a century. It is the left over by-product of coal processing and distillation. There are thousands of compounds in coal tar, and only a fraction of these are identified. For this reason, it is unlikely that coal tar would be approved by the FDA if presented for approval for new drug status *today*. In any case, coal tar is grandfathered in – it has been a medication longer than the FDA has existed. Before corticosteroids were first recognized or synthesized for use in inflammatory skin diseases, coal tar was there to help ease the itch. Some of my older professors originally practiced in the *pre-corticosteroid* era and were very adept at the use of coal tar compounds for skin therapy. Coal tar preparations appear to exert their anti-psoriasis benefits by interfering with DNA and thus slowing down skin cell growth and turnover. The long-term result is thinning of the psoriatic plaques.

How is Coal Tar Used?

Coal tar is found in dozens of over-the-counter psoriasis and dandruff shampoos, as well as creams, gels and bath additives. Compound pharmacists can mix crude coal tar (a black, thick paste) or coal tar solution (a 20% alcohol-based liquid) with all sorts of bases, including steroid creams and ointments. One effective remedy for hand and foot psoriasis is a compound of a steroid with 5% coal tar solution and 2% salicylic acid which a pharmacist can mix up with a prescription from your doctor.

What is Psoriasis?

Coal tar is often used in combination with phototherapy, as it sensitizes the skin to ultraviolet radiation. Care should be taken in avoiding excess sun exposure when using coal tar shampoos and other preparations.

Is Coal Tar Dangerous?

With many unknown ingredients, the question is not too easy to answer definitively. However, 5% or greater coal tar is classified as a carcinogen (cancer-causing agent) by the World Health Organization's International Agency for Research on Cancer. In this regard, it is in the same category as methoxsalen (used in PUVA therapy for psoriasis) and solar radiation, two other forms of psoriasis treatment. Alcoholic beverages and tobacco also qualify in this category.

There are not too many over-the-counter products that carry the full 5% crude coal tar concentration considered carcinogenic by the WHO, however California law is much more strict in this regard and considers even 0.5 coal tar dangerous enough to require a warning on a product's label . The FDA, in contrast, considers 0.5 to 5% OTC coal tar preparations safe for psoriasis, and there is really no evidence linking these weaker preparations to an increased risk of cancer. Although coal tar compounds have been found in the urine of users of an experimental tar-based shampoo, the concentration of coal tar used was around 100 times greater than that of common OTC shampoos.

Still Useful in Many Regards

For the most part, worries about coal tar are probably overblown. It has several merits, including very low cost and absence of steroids (and therefore steroid-related side effects). Typically it is left on for about two hours and rinsed off.

What is Psoriasis?

This short contact type of therapy helps to prevent staining of clothing and fabrics often seen with use of coal tar.

Further Reading:

Good 'ol Coal Tar Whips Dovonex! Coal tar is old, older than John McCain even, but that doens't mean its not still very useful. In fact a recent study of a novel coal tar preparation proved better than Calcipotriene in clearing psoriasis – only the coal tar patients achieved a PASI 75. Good work coal tar!

What is Psoriasis?

Section 7

Chinese Herbs for Psoriasis

A Scientific Look at the Use of Chinese Herbs for Psoriasis

Traditional Chinese medicine (TCM), including the use of Chinese herbs for psoriasis, is considered an alternative treatment in the West. But for a billion or more Chinese, it's a mainstream treatment option.

Traditional Therapies: Does Modern Science Deem Them Useful?

Traditional Chinese medicine relies heavily on herbal treatments as medications, including the use of Chinese herbs for psoriasis. Some herbal treatments have been studied in clinical and laboratory trials and the effects documented. Others have been linked to toxicities, especially liver toxicity.

An Herb That Can Stop Skin Cell Growth?

On at least a theoretical basis, *Radix Rubiae* – through its ability to prevent the growth of skin cells – may be useful in psoriasis. Scientists discovered the anti-proliferative activity of this herb while screening over 60 traditional anti-psoriatic Chinese herbs in the laboratory.

An Herbal Bath as a Treatment?

Many studies of TCM are published in Chinese medical literature. As such, access to this data for those who cannot read Chinese is limited. One more recent study published in Chinese had an English abstract with an overview of the methods and results. Over 100 psoriasis patients were studied. All subjects were treated with narrow-band UVB phototherapy, but in half the light treatment was preceded by a bath in an herbal concoction called *Yuyin Recipe*.

During the 8-week trial, those treated with the herbal bath had a greater reduction in their PASI scores, experienced fewer side effects, and needed a lower dose of ultraviolet light to achieve clearing of their psoriasis.

An abstract is just a snapshot of what's presented in a full study, so it offers only limited insight into a clinical trial such as this. Many facts not mentioned could be buried in the original Chinese language text.

What Does This Mean for You?
I'm going to venture a guess that you're not an expert in the use of Chinese herbs. I'll also bet that your corner store's herb section is limited to mint, thyme and the like. So, it would not be simple to try and replicate the above trial for personal use. An expert in TCM who is familiar with the specific Yuyin Recipe and able to review the original article for exactly how it was used would be needed.

Even if you can get your hands on Chinese herbs, you should not experiment with their use – especially in conjunction with any kind of ultraviolet light therapy. Many herbs are known to cause increased sensitivity to sunlight, and their use may result in unexpected burning with natural or artificial sunlight exposure.

"Natural" does not imply safe; several patients taking Chinese herbs have suffered liver toxicity, including at least one case of fatal liver damage. In addition, Chinese herbs, like most traditional medicines, are not as strictly regulated by the FDA as modern (allopathic) drugs are.

There indeed *may* be effective compounds in the complex herbal concoctions that make up TCM recipes. But figuring out what compounds may be having the positive affect, and whether or not these results are solid enough to be seen time and time again, requires more stringently-controlled and large studies that – to date – just don't exist.

Will eating curry help my psoriasis?

Question: Will eating curry help my psoriasis?

Answer:
There are some anecdotes of people who saw improvement in their psoriasis by eating a diet, which contained a lot of curry. Is there any scientific evidence to support this? Curry is the generic name for spicy gravy-laced culinary dishes from Asia made with the brightly colored herb (curcuma longa). There are some laboratory studies, which show that specific compounds found in this herb (called "curcuminoids") have anti-inflammatory properties. Specifically, these compounds seem to block TNF-alpha, much like the powerful biologic drugs we use to treat psoriasis. So is curry "nature's biologic" and can it help treat psoriasis?

Unfortunately, and anecdotes of a few lucky people aside, there are no good clinical studies demonstrating a beneficial effect of curry on psoriasis. In fact, a large Phase II clinical trial, which was completed in 2007 and published this year, found that the response to curcumin was no greater than a placebo. This was a very small trial; however, and a larger trial was suggested. Two people in the study did achieve a PASI 75, which although quite remarkable, was attributed to the natural course of the disease by the study authors. One criticism of the study would be the relatively small dose of curcuminoids

What is Psoriasis?

used, i.e. 4.5 grams daily. Since these compounds are very poorly absorbed by the digestive tract, a much larger quantity may be needed to provide for any sort of systemic treatment effect. Doses as high as 12 grams daily (nearly 3 times those used in the psoriasis trial) have been shown to be safe for prolonged periods of time. A smaller, uncontrolled clinical trial, using higher doses, saw some benefit from curcumin in several diseases, including psoriasis.

So what's the final verdict? I'm afraid it's not in yet. With no *good* clinical trial data either way, it's hard to recommend supplementation with curcumin as a treatment for psoriasis. I do continue to recommend that everyone, whether they have psoriasis or not, enjoy curry dishes just as much as they want!

Further Reading:

Some Curry a Day Keeps Psoriasis Away? I was intrigued by this blurb about a psoriasis patient who got better through the use of tumeric. Tumeric is an herb (sometimes called Curcumin) used in curry dishes. What's so interesting about this particular herb is that has been shown to have some anti-TNF alpha activity not too unlike some of the biologic drugs used for psoriasis. Seems this herb has caught the attention of researchers too. The University of Pennsylvania is currently recruiting patients for a study using curcuminoids (compounds from Curry) for the treatment of psoriasis. This is a phase II study meaning any clinical application is years away. Meanwhile don't be a stranger to your neighborhood Indian restaurant!

Indigo Plant Ointment for Psoriasis In a study out of China published in the Archives of Dermatology, scientists used an ointment compounded from Indigo plant extract to reduce the

---

redness and scaling of psoriasis. The ointment itself is apparently a bit smelly and temporarily stains the skin. However, no medical side effects were noted during the twelve-week study.

Can Olive Oil Help Psoriasis?

Many proponents of nutritional therapies for various diseases recognize that different types of oils may have varying effects on the body. One difference among types of oils is that some seem to promote inflammation while others are anti-inflammatory or neutral in this regard.

Recently I came across an article on using an olive oil supplement for the treatment of psoriasis. While such studies are not very reliable due to their small size and usually poor design they may shed some light on directions for future investigations. Most of the time however, such claims amount to little more than the promises of snake oil salesmen

Green Tea Shows Early Promise for Psoriasis in Animal Study

Researchers at the Medical College of Georgia found that green tea helped to reduce the rapid growth of skin cells, a key feature of Psoriasis. They studied green tea in rodents genetically predisposed to develop Psoriasis-like skin changes. Green tea may help regulate expression of a protein called Caspase-14, which is involved in cell cycle regulation (the process of cell growth and reproduction). Although this data is interesting, the absolute role of diet in Psoriasis remains very poorly understood.

What is Psoriasis?

Section 8

Psoriasis Treatment Overview

So Many Options

Psoriasis has more treatment options than most skin diseases. You can be treated *externally*, with creams and similar topical medications, as well as *internally*, with pills or injections. For more difficult or severe psoriasis, you may wish to consult with a dermatologist.

Physical treatments, such as natural or artificial sunlight (phototherapy), are also extensively used.

Finding a treatment or combination of treatments that's just right and effective for *you* may take some trial and error, and sometimes the logistics (such as the stickiness of topicals or the frequent office visits required by phototherapy) can be daunting. Despite this, you can expect significant clearing of your skin with appropriate treatment over time.

- **Topical Treatments**

Psoriasis treatment is available both over-the-counter and by prescription. Topical preparations are available as creams, ointments, lotions, oils, foams, and tapes, make treating any body part possible. When these fail, or the amount of skin to be treated is too great (typically >10% of the body), then systemic treatments are recommended.

What is Psoriasis?

- **Systemic Treatments**

Systemic treatments are those medications that treat the whole body, rather than just the affected area. For psoriasis, this includes pills and injections.

Prescription pills for psoriasis include methotrexate and Soriatane. Although studied for psoriasis, other pills (such as sulfasalazine and hydroxyurea) are seldom used, but may be recommended to specific patients. Potent immunosuppressive drugs, such as cyclosporine and 6-mercaptopurine based drugs, play a role in psoriasis treatment for very select patients.

Injectable biologics are the new kids on the block, but they have made a tremendous impact on the way we treat moderate to severe psoriasis. Now, with as little as twice monthly injections at home, psoriasis patients can be relatively disease-free. There are many biologics to choose from. Like all medications, these too have side effects and require monitoring by the physician to observe for complications. Nevertheless, they represent a quantum leap in therapy and a big change in the life of many patients with otherwise debilitating psoriasis.

- **Physical Treatments**

Phototherapy using ultraviolet light can be very effective for psoriasis. Previously, UVB and PUVA (UVA exposure after ingestion of a sun-sensitizing pill) were the most common forms of light therapy. A newer treatment called narrow-band UVB (NB-UVB) seems to work at least as well as these if not better, and with fewer side effects. The latest equipment uses laser to deliver NB-UVB with pinpoint accuracy. Heliotherapy uses the

What is Psoriasis?

sun as a source of natural ultraviolet radiation to treat psoriasis. Treatment with light is not appropriate for every patient.

Topical Psoriasis Treatments

Creams, ointments, gels, and more
Most patients with psoriasis covering only a small portion of their bodies can usually get their condition under control with topical treatment -- creams, gels, or other medications applied directly to the skin. There are several different types of topical treatments available.

Corticosteroids
The most common drugs used in a topical preparation are corticosteroids. (These steroids are not to be confused with the type of steroids that make you grow muscles.) The mildest of these, hydrocortisone is available over-the-counter in a 1% strength. Psoriasis, however, is often too stubborn to treat with OTC hydrocortisone alone. Cortisone creams come in many strengths (classes), and higher strengths require a prescription. The stronger the cortisone, the lower the class. Class 1 steroids are *exponentially* stronger than class 7 steroids.

Strong steroid creams have side effects that are not to be underestimated. They can cause stretch marks to develop in closed areas, such as the armpits and groin, and tend to thin the skin over time. Covering large areas of the body with strong steroids can suppress the body's natural cortisol production, reducing your ability to cope with stresses like infection, injury or surgery. Always ask your doctor *exactly* where you *are and are not* supposed to apply any topical.

Non-Steroids
We can lump anything that's not a steroid into this group.

What is Psoriasis?

- Immune modulating drugs, such as Protopic (tacrolimus) and Elidel (pimecrolimus), reduce inflammation without the side effects of steroids.
- Vitamin D-derived Dovonex (calcipotriene) and Vectical normalize cell growth.
- Tazorac (tazarotene) is a retinoid (vitamin-A like) drug which normalizes cell growth and maturation.
- Anthralin works by slowing down the rapid skin cell growth seen in psoriasis.

The side effects of the non-steroids are typically less worrisome than their steroid cousins, but they are also usually slower acting or less potent.

Not Just Greasy Ointments Anymore
Topical drugs for psoriasis come in a dizzying variety, including ointments for dry areas, creams for moist areas, watery liquids, oils, gels and foams for hairy areas, tapes for thickened areas, and sprays for large areas. Whatever area of your body you need to treat, you can be sure there is a product designed just for it.

Topical Corticosteroids for Psoriasis

So Many Choices for So Many Body Parts

Seven Different Potencies
When we talk about steroids for psoriasis, we mean anti-inflammatory corticosteroids. Topical corticosteroids are divided into seven different categories based upon strength. The mildest of these, class 7, includes over-the-counter hydrocortisone 1%. The strongest, class 1, consist of the "big gun" steroid creams, such as clobetasole.

What is Psoriasis?

Why More Isn't Better
Class 1 steroids are not just a little stronger than class 7, they are *exponentially* stronger and, therefore, can cause more side effects. Using a too-strong steroid on the face can lead to acne, rosacea and the development of little red blood vessels called telangiectasia. The eyes can be damaged by strong steroids, leading to glaucoma and cataracts.

In the groin and armpits, stronger classes of steroid can cause large red stretch marks to develop, which are usually permanent. Also, continuous use of strong steroids on the same exact areas leads to thinning of the skin (atrophy), which can also be permanent.

Lastly, covering large areas of your body with potent steroid creams can lead to systemic absorption and loss of the body's ability to make its own natural cortisol. An overabundance of cortisone-related drugs can produce *an exogenous adrenal insufficiency* state.

For all the above reasons, I usually try to use the *least potent* steroid which will actually get the job done choosing carefully for variable such as patient age, location of psoriasis and amount of body surface to be treated.

More Than Grease
One of my patients used to always come to the office for refills: "I'm out of *grease*" he'd say. But topical corticosteroids come in all sorts of vehicles:

- Ointments (petrolatum-based "grease")
- Creams (lighter and less greasy, much nicer to use on the face, groin or armpits)
- Oils (for whole-body treatment or for overnight scalp treatment)

All About Psoriasis for Psoriasis Patients Page 77

- Gels (completely absorb and non-greasy, great for hairy areas)
- Foams (easy to spread and also good for scalp and hairy areas)
- Tapes (for thicker plaques such as elbows and knees)

In general, for a given active ingredient, ointments will be more potent than creams (but also more messy). Foams have proven to be very effective in that they tend to penetrate to deeper layers of the skin than other vehicles. Hence, a slightly less potent active ingredient may give more benefit if used as a foam.

Taclonex (Calcipotriene and Betamethasone Dipropionate)

Dovonex (calcipotriene) for psoriasis has been available for over a decade. Altough effective for some patients, the drug is notoriously slow in achieving clearing of psoriasis. Almost as soon as it was released, doctors were using it in combination with corticosteroid creams to help speed up results.

One difficulty with these combinations is that the calcipotriene ingredient was not stable at the same pH as the corticosteroid ingredient, hence applying both creams together *reduced* the effectiveness. This necessitated in all sorts of treatment schedules such as Dovonex weekdays and corticosteroid creams weekends or Dovonex in the morning and corticosteroid creams at night. The stability problem has been overcome and now both drugs have been combined into a single, once-daily ointment called *Taclonex*.

Taclonex is indicated for the treatment of psoriasis vulgaris in adults. It shouldn't be applied to the face, armpits or groin because it does contain a potent corticosteroid ingredient. The once-daily, as-needed dosing schedule is more convenient than most other topical medications[5] for psoriasis.

Tazorac (Tazorotene)

A Topical Retinoid for Psoriasis

What is Tazarotene?
Tazarotene is a vitamin A-derived drug that is part of a class of drugs called retinoids. Unlike the more famous retinoid drug, Retin-A, tazarotene can improve psoriasis. It is available under the brand name Tazorac.

How is it Used
Tazorac comes in two strengths, 0.05 and 0.1%, and is available as both a cream and a gel. The 0.1% gel is the strongest version; your dermatologist can help you decide which one is right for you. This medication is applied once daily. It can take 2 to 12 weeks for you to see maximum improvement. Tazorac can be combined with topical steroids, Dovonex, phototherapy, and other treatments. It can be somewhat drying, and using a moisturizer in addition to the drug is usually recommended.

Tazorac can be used in the morning, as no messy residue is left behind. This is especially helpful for those with hand psoriasis. At night, a messier ointment can be used. Tazorac is one of the only topical psoriasis medications that may help fingernail psoriasis.

Dovonex (Calcipotriene)

A Vitamin D Cream for Psoriasis

What is Calcipotriene?
Calcipotriene was created to fill the need of a drug that would suppress rapid skin cell growth (as seen in psoriasis) without upsetting normal calcium metabolism, like natural vitamin D does. It is available as a cream and scalp liquid under the brand name Dovonex. A combination ointment of calcipotriene with a steroid cream is marketed under the name Taclonex. Dovonex works slowly and the cream version is relatively weak. Studies have shown it to be as effective as a strong steroid cream. Nevertheless, it has a valuable role in treating psoriasis in that it has none of the side effects typically expected with the prolonged use of steroid creams. It is sometimes not recommended for use on the face since it can cause redness.   A newer drug called Vectical is similar to Dovonex, but can be used on the face and groin without causing redness. Vectical has more or less replaced Dovonex as the main vitamin D drug for psoriasis.

How is it Used?
Dovonex can be applied twice daily, and results are usually seen around 4 to 6 weeks into treatment. It can be used continuously and is safe for patients who have psoriasis on up to 20% of their body. It can be combined with other treatments, including topical steroids and phototherapy. Vectical is applied once daily.

Zithronal RR (anthralin): Topical Cream for Psoriasis

Topical Anthralin is Still Useful in Psoriasis Treatment
Anthralin is one of the original psoriasis topical medications. Decades ago, generic anthralin paste was applied thickly to plaques of psoriasis and then dusted with a powder. The treatment was effective, but also messy. It was usually performed only in hospitals or psoriasis day treatment centers for this reason.

Such intensive psoriasis therapies have generally fallen to the wayside in favor of the more convenient treatments we have at our disposal today. Nevertheless, anthralin is still a useful drug, especially in its newest iteration, Zithronal RR cream.

Zithronal RR: Anthralin Reincarnated
Zithronal RR is a new (and at present, only) version of anthralin. It is a timed-release cream, meaning the active ingredient is very slowly released into the skin. This helps minimizes the irritation that was sometimes seen with generic anthralin in the past. The instructions for use have also been designed to reduce side effects, such as irritation and skin staining (also drawbacks to traditional anthralin treatment).

Convenient Use of Psoriatec
Unlike previous versions of anthralin, Zithronal RR can be relatively convenient to use by following instructions for what's known as short contact anthralin therapy (SCAT).

Here's how it works:
It is usually recommended that patients apply the cream to the affected areas about 30 minutes before taking a shower. Patients with guttate psoriasis covering most of their body can

cover large areas, even normal skin, as the application time is too brief to cause irritation to surrounding healthy skin. Once time is up, a cool water shower is used to wash away the cream. This rinse removes the cream without activating the time-released drug, another measure designed to reduce inflammation and irritation. A normal warm water shower with soap is then taken.

How Soon Can You See Results?
Anthralin (in any form) is not a drug for people in a hurry. It can take weeks or months to get good results. Still, using the drug does have its upsides:

- There are no steroids in anthralin.
- It will not thin the skin or cause stretch marks.
- It is not as costly as some of the newer kids on the block, such as Taclonex.
- It sometimes works great when nothing else seems to.
- You can apply Zithronal RR to the scalp before shampooing to treat tough psoriasis scales and plaques.

As with any drug, you should discuss and weigh the risks and rewards of using a medication with your doctor before use.

Protopic and Elidel for Psoriasis

Strength Without Steroids
Here's a dilemma: You need to treat psoriasis on an area where strong topical steroids may be a problem, but milder corticosteroids are ineffective. What do you do? One easy solution is to use a non-steroid topical medication. However, many of these, like Dovonex or Zithronal RR are typically too irritating to use on sensitive facial or groin skin. For a solution, we have to look outside the list of FDA-approved psoriasis

What is Psoriasis?

drugs and utilize some drugs used and approved for eczema. Using an approved drug for an unapproved use is called "off-label" use and it's not only perfectly legal, its actually quite common in dermatology practice. The drugs I'm referring to are Protopic (tacrolimus) and Elidel (pimecrolimus).

Protopic is an ointment which can be useful for psoriasis of the face and groin. One unusual side effect of Protopic is that areas treated become red upon ingestion of alcohol -- something which patients may have brought to their attention at a dinner party if they are not warned of this beforehand. Elidel works like Protopic, but its cream base is less greasy and perhaps a bit more comfortable (although it may not be quite as effective for this condition). Both drugs are excellent for inverse psoriasis of the skin folds. They also both may cause a bit of mild stinging with initial use. Several years after their release, both drugs received a "black box" warning regarding risks of infection or malignancy. The American Academy of Dermatology and others have gone on record with the position that the drugs are indeed safe when used appropriately.

Whether or not off-label use of these drugs is right for you is a decision you and your dermatologist have to make together. At times, insurance companies are reluctant to cover the use of these relatively expensive drugs when cheaper steroids are available. However, a letter from your dermatologist indicating the specific need for a non-steroid drug in a given circumstance may get the drug approved.

Vectical, the vitamin D based ointment can is another non-steroid choice for use in sensitive areas like the face, underarms or groin.

What is Psoriasis?

All Body Parts are Not Equal:

Psoriasis Treatment Options Vary
It's important to consider several factors when selecting a psoriasis treatment for a specific part of the body. Each has its own set of charactertics that may make one treatment option more desirable than another.

Genital Psoriasis
Genital psoriasis is relatively common; however undue patient reluctance to discuss this problem may delay diagnosis or result in the wrong treatment being used. It is vitally important that patients don't *assume* that a cream prescribed for hands or elbows is safe when used on another body part like genitals or face. In this regard, the skin of this region is already thin which can promote excessive absorption of medications as well as further thinning or *atrophy* if overly strong steroid creams are applied. An excellent choice for psoriasis of the genitals includes hydrocortisone/iodoquinol cream (previously known as the branded product Vytone).

Psoriasis of the Palms and Soles

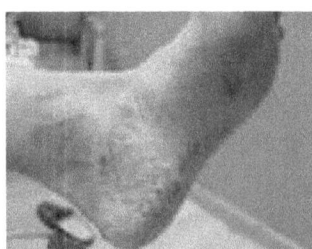

©New Paradigm Dermatology, PL

Psoriasis of the palms and soles, *palmoplantar psoriasis*, requires extra potent medication due to the thickness of the skin being treated. Psoriasis in these areas is often rather scaly and extra thick compared to other body parts. Ingredients de-

What is Psoriasis?

signed to dissolve flakes and enhance penetration of the medications can be compounded into topical creams and ointments to make them more effective for hands and feet. One effective combination, which can be made by prescription, includes a strong topical steroid (such as clobetasole) along with a salicylic acid and coal tar solution. Although messy and smelly, this combination is quite effective for thick, stubborn palmoplantar psoriasis.

Skin Fold Psoriasis

Also known as *flexural or inverse psoriasis,* psoriasis of skin folds is frequently mistaken for yeast or fungus infections due to the locations involved (armpits, under breast and between the thighs in the groin). Because psoriasis is inflammatory and not infectious, a straightforward antifungal cream usually has little effect on flexural psoriasis. However since yeast can trigger or aggravate the condition, it is not surprising that one of the most effective creams for inverse psoriasis includes a mild steroid mixed with ketoconazole, an antifungal ingredient. As with genital psoriasis, one worry with flexural psoriasis is atrophy and even stretch marks resulting from overly strong steroid creams being applied here.

Scalp Psoriasis

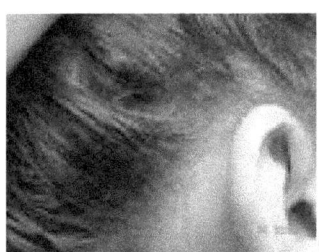
©*New Paradigm Dermatology, PL*

Treatment of scalp psoriasis is difficult due to the inability to apply medications directly onto a hairy scalp, as well as the

What is Psoriasis?

mess of using greasy ointments there. Two solutions are to use medicated shampoos (such as Pentrax or Sebulex) and non-greasy medications, such as Luxiq or Olux foams. When flaking is severe, it is sometimes necessary to apply a medicated oil (such as Dermasmoothe FS) at night and wash it out in the morning. The medications mentioned here require a prescription from your doctor, but the shampoos are available over the counter.

Facial Psoriasis

Psoriasis of the face, like that of the skin folds or genitals requires a gentle medication to avoid side effects. In addition to the thinning and stretch marks seen with strong steroids in other areas, these medications can easily cause acne or rosacea to break out when used on the face. In addition, strong steoids used for long periods of time around the eyes may promote cataracts or glaucoma. In many instances, over the counter hydrocortisone 1% cream is adequate for mild psoriasis of the face.

Section 9

Methotrexate

Tried and True Psoriasis Treatment Since 1958:
Methotrexate (MTX) interferes with the normal metabolism of folate, a B vitamin. It inhibits the growth of cells. Cells that grow rapidly, such as skin cells in psoriasis, are more susceptible to MTX than normal cells.

A major drawback to the use of methotrexate is that users must undergo a liver biopsy every few years (after each 1,500 mg total cumulative dose) to check for liver disease (cirrhosis). The real and perceived risks of this procedure have been a factor in the success of the newer biologic drugs, which do not share this requirement.

Who Should Take This Drug?:
Methotrexate is recommended for those who have psoriasis over a good portion of their body. It should be used when other treatments, such as phototherapy or acetretin, have already failed. It is also a very effective drug against psoriatic arthritis. In these instances, MTX can be considered a first-line treatment choice.

Methotrexate is a very effective weapon against difficult psoriasis, such as exfoliative erythroderma (where the entire body turns red) and generalized pustular psoriasis.

Which Patients Should Avoid This Drug?:
Methotrexate should be avoided or used with extreme caution in patients with current or planned pregnancy,

What is Psoriasis?

alcoholism, hepatitis, cirrhosis, renal failure, immunodeficiency and blood disorders.

What are the Side Effects of Methotrexate?:
Methotrexate is a relatively toxic drug, and care must be taken to monitor for problems, such as oral ulcerations, bone marrow suppression, lymphoma, birth defects, sun sensitivity, and lung, liver, and kidney toxicity. The more serious of these, however, are relatively rare with the low doses of methotrexate used to treat psoriasis.

Soriatane (acetretin)

A Vitamin A "Drug" for Psoriasis:
Soriatane (acetretin) is a laboratory derivative of vitamin A (retinoic acid), a class of drugs known as *retinoids*. Doctors have known that megadoses of vitamin A can minimize thickness and scaliness of the skin in psoriasis. One topical retinoid for psoriasis is Tazorac.

Unfortunately, the systemic doses of vitamin A needed to treat psoriasis are very toxic and can cause liver damage and death. Soriatane reduces (but does not eliminate) the unwanted toxicity of vitamin A while enhancing the desirable effects on abnormally thick and scaly skin. The result is a strong and effective oral psoriasis treatment.

Who Should Take This Drug?: Soriatane is a treatment option for persons with severe psoriasis, for example when it involves greater than 10% of the body's surface area. It is also effective for another severe type of psoriasis called pustular psoriasis.

What is Psoriasis?

Which Patients Should Avoid This Drug?: Soriatane is not recommended for women who may become pregnant because it can cause severe birth defects. The risk of birth defects lasts many years after stopping the drug. For this reason, the drug is mainly used in men and post-menopausal women (or women who have undergone surgical sterilization).

What are the Side Effects of Soriatane?: There are some bothersome side effects such as dry skin and lips that are routinely seen with the use of Soriatane. Other side effects such as joint pain and hair loss are less frequent. More serious side effects such as increased blood lipids or abnormal liver function blood tests may require discontinuation of treatment. Patients using Soriatane should not donate blood since this blood could end up being used in a pregnant patient.

Cyclosporine

A Fast and Powerful Pill for Psoriasis:
Cyclosporine is generally considered a quick-acting and powerful psoriasis treatment drug. Because of cyclosporine's relatively risky side-effects profile, newer safer drugs have made the use of cyclosporine less popular. There are however patients for whom this drug is quite useful.

Who Should Take This Drug?:
Patients with severe psoriasis can use cyclosporine, preferably for the short term. Examples include those transitioning to a slower-acting but safer medicine as well as patients who are flaring or failing another treatment who need help fast.

What is Psoriasis?

Which Patients Should Avoid This Drug?:
Since it is an immunity-suppressing drug, patients with serious infections or cancer should avoid cyclosporine. It should also be avoided if you have hypertension or kidney disease. Caution should be used if you're taking other medications since it can interact with many commonly used drugs.

What are the Side Effects of Cyclosporine?:
The serious side effects that usually limit the use of cyclosporine to short periods include hypertension and kidney damage. Less serious side effects include overgrowth of gum tissue (gingival hyperplasia) and excess hair growth (hirsutism).

Psorizide Forte, a Homeopathic Prescription Drug for Psoriasis

A Homeopathic Prescription Drug for Psoriasis: Psorizide Forte is an oral medication developed by a dermatologist for psoriasis. Initially, it was entered into the new drug application process for the FDA for allopathic drugs. It was realized afterwards that the ingredients used had been "grandfathered in" to the approved pharmacopeia for homeopathic drugs and so the drug was entered into the marketplace as a homeopathic drug instead.

Who Should Take This Drug?: Psorizide Forte is indicated for mild to severe psoriasis. This is not a commonly prescribed medication for many dermatologists. It may be useful in patients who are not suitable candidates for other systemic medications for psoriasis, or who can not afford the sometimes costly required laboratory monitoring needed with stronger medications.

What is Psoriasis?

Which Patients Should Avoid This Drug?: Contraindications to Psorizide Forte include the concurrent use of certain sedatives and sleeping pills as well as hypersensitivity (allergy) to the ingredients (nickel sulphate, fumaric acid and potassium bromide). Nickel is a relatively common contact allergen. People who develop rashes when contacting nickel should start with a very low dose and increase slowly to allow desensitization to occur. Those with serious nickel allergy should avoid this drug. This drug should be used with caution in kidney disease. It is pregnancy category C and its safety in pregnancy has not been evaluated.

What are the Side Effects of This Drug?: There are no significant side effects to Psorizide Forte other than the possibility of hypersensitivity (allergic reaction) to the ingredients.

Seldom Used Drugs for Psoriasis

Before biologic drugs were invented, there were a few drugs that were used for more severe cases of psoriasis, typically when more standard drugs such as methothrexate or Soriatane didn't work. For example:

Cyclosporine
This compound is a protein originally isolated from a soil fungus. It prevents the activation of T-cells that cause inflammation in psoriasis and other diseases. Cyclosporine is still used today quite commonly in organ transplant patients; in fact, it was by accidentally observing improvement in psoriasis in transplant patients that its effectiveness in psoriasis was first discovered. The newer topical drugs Elidel and Protopic are of the same drug class as cyclosporine and work in the same manner.

What is Psoriasis?

Cyclosporine is a very fast acting drug which can clear psoriasis in 8 weeks or so. But, unfortunately, the remission times are rather short requiring continuous or frequent short courses of the drug. Because of the kidney toxicity and blood pressure problems caused by cyclosporine, it is not used as frequently in psoriasis as other drugs.

Hydroxyurea

Hydroxyurea was first used for psoriasis in 1970 as an alternative to methotrexate. It is more commonly used by hematologists in the treatment of blood disorders. Hydroxyurea works by preventing the synthesis of DNA, a necessary step in cell duplication which is typically markedly increased in psoriasis. Hydroxyurea is only a moderately effective drug with multiple toxicities which requires extensive monitoring, for this reason it is seldom used for psoriasis.

Sulfasalazine

This sulfa-based anti-inflammatory drug is used as a second-line agent in many inflammatory diseases including inflammatory bowel disease, rheumatoid arthritis and ankylosing spondylitis. It appears to work by decreasing an inflammatory chemical called 5-lipoxygenase. The few studies done on this drug in psoriasis show that only about half of patients respond well to sulfasalazine. Sulfaszalazine has frequent side effects such as headache, nausea and rashes, which many times lead to discontinuation of the drug before any significant benefit has been seen.

Like methotrexate, sulfasalazine can also be useful for psoriatic arthritis. It is sometimes useful as a third-line drug after the other psoriasis pills (methotrexate and Soriatane) and is considerably less expensive than the more effective and more popular biologics. Extensive blood monitoring is required with this drug, although there is little long-term toxicity, such as increased risk of malignancy or infection, seen with some of the other psoriasis systemic medications. There are other seldom used drugs in psoriasis out there, but they are the *really* seldom used ones and as such have not been included here.

Psoriasis Treatments That are Fast

When Time is of the Essence

Speed is only one characteristic of a drug which may be of importance -- safety, side effects, cost, and medical reasons why a certain drug can't be used are just a few of the many others. But when time is of the essence, a faster drug may be just what the doctor ordered. Imagine that you're a month away from a cruise and you want to relax by the pool, but feel uncomfortable due to a breakout of psoriasis. That's just the type of situation when you want to get cleared up, *fast*. Here are a few medications with very rapid onset of action and clearing ability to consider:

Clobex Spray

Clobex spray is really just clobetasole, a potent corticosteroid, in a spray vehicle. A vehicle is the base in which a drug is mixed; the vehicle *delivers* the drug to the skin just like UPS vehicles deliver products to your house. Something about using the drug with the spray vehicle makes it faster than other vehicles. In studies, 8 out of 10 patients with moderate-to-severe plaque-type psoriasis were clear or almost clear after just four weeks of treatment. That's the good news. The bad news is four weeks is the maximum time that you can safely use this drug. After that, you'll need to switch to something else.

What is Psoriasis?

I like to use Clobex spray as an adjunct to a slower-acting, but perhaps safer, long-term drug just to initiate a rapid clearing. For example, Clobex spray during the first month of a course of Soriatane or a biologic may give a faster response than the latter drugs alone. After the first month, the Clobex spray is discontinued by which time the slower acting drug has had a chance to kick in.

Side effects of Clobex spray are those of topical corticosteroids including thinning of the skin, stretch marks and faltering of natural production of the hormone cortisol. With the short course approved, these problems are less likely to occur. Clobex spray is not for children, nor for use on the face, on underarms or the groin area.

Cyclosporine

Cyclosporine is more commonly used for organ transplant patients as an anti-rejection drug but is sometimes used in psoriasis. Neoral is a brand of cyclosporine available in both pill and oral-liquid form. Cyclosporine is effective rapidly for psoriasis, with some improvement noted within the first week in many patients. The side effects of the drug are very dose-dependent. In other words, the higher doses that lead to rapid improvement also result in a quicker onset of side effects such as kidney toxicity and hypertension. Psoriasis patients with a history of PUVA treatment have a higher risk of developing skin cancer while using cyclosporine. Biologics, which appear to have a safer risk to benefit ratio compared to cyclosporine, have more or less supplanted this drug for psoriasis in most patients.

Humira

Humira is generally considered the fastest of the lot. It also produces good clearing with more patients being 90% cleared

What is Psoriasis?

than the competing biologic drugs. Humira was previously approved for psoriatic arthritis at a dose of one injection every other week. When the drug was approved for psoriasis, a dose was added which essentially called for two additional doses of the drug over the first week of treatment. This change greatly accelerated the improvement seen in psoriasis versus the previous dosing schedule.

Humira may increase the risk of severe infection or malignancy. Fortunately, as more and more data comes to light, these risks are appearing to be less worrisome than originally anticipated some years ago.

Better Data Would be Helpful
Although the above mentioned drugs *seem* fast, few studies comparing them to *other drugs* have been done. Drug companies rarely do comparison studies of their drugs versus another (rather they like to test versus a placebo). So for the time being it's more a matter of *perceived speed* than hard, cold facts.

Further Reading:

Antibiotics for Guttate Psoriasis
Sometimes guttate psoriasis responds to antibiotics. The rational is that the guttate flare was triggered by a strep infection, possibly a strep throat. Researchers in Bulgaria tested the antibiotic rifampin in 52 patients with guttate psoriasis. Over 60 days they noted about 2/3 improvement in PASI scores. The improvement was similar whether or not the patients had a strep infection. Their hypothesis is that in this instance, the antibiotic rifampin may have acted as a mild immunosuppressant.

What is Psoriasis?

Folic Acid Helpful for Patients Taking Methotrexate

Methotrexate is a commonly used psoriasis and psoriatic arthritis drug. Liver toxicity is a primary concern with the use of this drug and blood tests and even liver biopsies are often used to monitor for signs of toxicity. An article published in the British Journal of Dermatology reviewed six studies where folic acid supplementation was used to combat methotrexate-induced liver toxidity. The study showed that folic acid reduced *short term* liver toxicity by over 30 percent. What was not evaluated was *long term* liver toxicity, which in its final form leads to cirrhosis of the liver.

I typically have methotrexate-treated patients take folic acid on the day or days they don't take their methotrexate. Other studies have mentioned less GI upset with folic acid supplementation. In any case, don't take the folic acid without discussing it with your doctor first, because taking it incorrectly may reduce the effectiveness of your methotrexate. Finally, with no good test or preventative measure to avoid fibrosis of the liver, I always have my methotrexate patients have a liver biopsy with every 1500mg total cummulative dose of methotrexate. For most patients, this is about 1-2 years of treatment.

Section 10

UVB and PUVA for Psoriasis

Artificial Sunlight for Your Skin

Although phototherapy equipment is classified as a device rather than a drug, such equipment is usually seen in a doctor's office or obtained with a doctor's prescription. For these reasons, phototherapy is listed here under "Psoriasis Drugs".

Experiments with ultraviolet light and psoriasis date back to the 1920s. Since then, ultraviolet light has become a standard treatment for extensive psoriasis and is referred to as phototherapy.

Ultraviolet light is a part of the *electromagnetic spectrum*. A complete review of the physics of the electromagnetic spectrum is well beyond the scope of this article. But suffice it to say that ultraviolet light is invisible to the naked eye, yet contains enough energy to both treat and/or burn the skin.

The sun produces ultraviolet light (UV). Three types of UV light are UVA, UVB and UVC. The effects of UVA are essentially therapeutic for psoriasis while producing minimal burning. UVB can be therapeutic but also can cause sunburn. UVC is used as germicidal light. For example, you may see UVC bulbs in restaurants, operating rooms or laboratories to kill airborne bacteria, but it does not help psoriasis.

Modern phototherapy relies upon use of a small portion of UVB that is termed "narrow-band" UVB (NB-UVB). This small subset of UVB is effective at treating the skin with less burning

What is Psoriasis?

potential than natural UVB rays. Phototherapy equipment can be ordered specifically with bulbs that emit only narrow-band UVB for both home and in-office, physician-directed treatments.

Taking a pill called psoralen can make the skin more susceptible to the effects of UVA. Psoralen plus UVA phototherapy (called PUVA) can be effective for psoriasis even when UVB fails. Oral psoralen can have side effects such as nausea and the sensitivity to UV for both skin and eyes remains in the body for about 24 hours after it is taken. That means you should wear sunscreen, hat, long sleeves and dark sunglasses the entire day of treatment. This makes the logistics of PUVA somewhat daunting.

Topical medicines such as coal tar are often used for UVB phototherapy to enhance its effectiveness, again by making the skin more sensitive to UV.

A typical course of NB-UVB works something like this:

1. patient is a candidate for systemic therapy (more than a cream) based upon severity of disease
2. other medical reasons prohibiting phototherapy are absent
3. patients medication list is reviewed for photosensitizing meds
4. patient is selected for phototherapy, the risks as well as benefits explained, and consent obtained
5. patient takes NB-UVB treatments 3 to 5 times weekly
6. dosage (time of exposure) to NB-UVB is typically increased each visit

7. after approximately one month, they usually show improvement
8. after approximately two months, many patients are clear of psoriasis
9. patient may elect to continue therapy once weekly to maintain their improvement, or spend time outdoors every weekend to expose their psoriasis to natural UV radiation to do the same.

Phototherapy is an effective treatment for patients with severe or extensive psoriasis where application of topical medicines is not practical or effective. There is limited or no internal side effects to phototherapy verus pills or injections. Care must be taken to avoid treating patients with medical reasons to avoid phototherapy such as medications which make them sensitive to sunlight.

Excimer Laser for Psoriasis

Pinpoint Accuracy for Treatment of Small, but Stubborn Psoriasis Plaques

Treatment with Light
Phototherapy means treatment with light. For decades, phototherapy generally relied upon surrounding the patient with full-length fluorescent light bulbs in a specially designed cabinet. In this way, the entire body could be treated with therapeutic ultraviolet light.

What is Psoriasis?

A Niche Treatment for Small Spots

Although generally effective, it can be somewhat troublesome to use phototherapy to treat small areas of the body. For example, what if someone just wanted their hands or feet treated? In these instances, a special booth with openings for the hands or feet can be used, sparing the rest of the body unnecessary exposure to ultraviolet light.

But what if you just have a few very stubborn plaques of psoriasis? Can you spot treat areas with ultraviolet light? The answer is yes and the tools used are special lasers called 308nm excimer lasers. This type of laser is specially designed to produce ultraviolet radiation at a very specific wavelength - 308 nanometers. This wavelength of ultraviolet light is highly effective at treating psoriasis. A nearly identical wavelength of light, 311nm is referred to as narrow band UVB (NB-UVB) but is only available using special fluorescent light bulbs in the aforementioned cabinets or booths. Excimer laser gives us the benefits of NB-UVB with the small treatment areas typically ascribed to laser treatments (for example, a particularly stubborn plaque of psoriasis on the elbow or knee).

Getting it Done

It usually takes about 10 to 15 treatments with the excimer laser to achieve substantial improvement in a plaque of psoriasis. One major advantage of excimer laser treatment is that remission times are generally much longer than treatments relying on topical creams.

Various brands of excimer laser equipment are now on the market. Medicare and most private insurance carriers will cover this treatment for suitable patients. If you live in a larger city or suburb, it is very likely that a dermatologist near you offers this treatment.

Who Should Avoid Light Therapy (Phototherapy and Heliotherapy)?

Light Therapies for Psoriasis Treatment are Not for Everyone
Phototherapy and heliotherapy are two treatments that may be recommended for the treatment of psoriasis. Both involve exposure to light.

While effective, some people should avoid excess ultraviolet radiation -- natural or synthetic -- for the treatment of their psoriasis. These people include:

- patients with light sensitive diseases, including but not limited to lupus or porphyria
- patients with a history of melanoma or invasive squamous cell carcinomas of the skin (skin cancer)
- Patients who have had their eyes' natural lenses removed due to cataracts, since the lens protects the retina against UV radiation
- women who are pregnant

Special care should be taken when using ultraviolet radiation to treat patients who have a history of basal cell carcinoma of the skin, arsenic exposure, or a history of prior x-ray therapy.

What is Psoriasis?

Further Reading:

Narrow Band UVB Phototherapy does not Cause Skin Cancer
Researchers in Scotland found no association between NB-UVB phototherapy and the development of squamous cell, basal cell or melanoma forms of skin cancer in a study involving over three thousand patients. This data should be quite reassuring to patients currently undergoing this form of treatment. They did find however, that patients who had also received PUVA in addition to NB-UVB had an increased risk of basal cell carcinoma.

Goeckerman Regimen Best for Patients with Higher IL-10 Levels to Start
Czech researchers looked at levels of an inflammatory cytokine called IL-10 in psoriasis patients before and after treatment with the Goeckerman Regimen. In this treatment regimen, patient with psoriasis are exposed to ultraviolet light after application of coal tar. According to the study, those patients with higher IL-10 levels before treatment reaped the most benefits. Such findings may allow for doctors to select which patients are best suited for this therapy.

Section 11

Choosing the Best Biologic for Your Psoriasis

Side Effects and Benefits of the Major Players
There are currently two main classes of biologic drugs for psoriasis: the ones that block a chemical called TNF-alpha such as Enbrel (etanercept), Remicade (infliximab) and Humira (adalimumab), and the one that blocks interleukins called Stelara (ustekinumab).

Arthritis
The TNF-alpha blocking drugs have the advantage of also treating psoriatic arthritis. The other types of biologics are not helpful in this regard.

Staying power
Some patients notice a diminution of the effectiveness of TNF-alpha blocking drugs over months to years, however this is not universal.

Convenience
The way that each drug is given varies and may play a role in deciding which one is best for you. Humira is given once every other week, Enbrel once or twice weekly and Stelara once quarterly. Enbrel and Humira are easy sub-cutaneous (shallow) self-administered drugs, much like insulin. A special pen-like device is used to self-inject the drugs and a needle is never actually seen. Stelara is also sub-cutaneous, but is administered every three months in the doctor's office. The drugs need to be refrigerated, which must be kept in mind for those

What is Psoriasis?

patients who travel frequently. Remicade is given as an IV in-
fusion in a doctor's office.

Special Benefits
Stelara is a weight-based biologic. In other words, heavier patients are injected with more drug. The other sub cutaneously
injected biologics listed here are dosed on a one-size-fits-all
basis. For this reason, heavier patients may in fact be under
dosed. This is an important consideration in view of the finding that obesity and psoriasis often go hand in hand.

Side Effects
It is not unusual to see local injection site reactions (redness
and tenderness) where the medications are injected into the
body. All the biologics affect the immune system, therefore
there is concern with all of them regarding serious infections
and malignancy. Many dermatologists now do a PPD test for
tuberculosis exposure before starting biologic drugs. Hepatitis
B exposure can be tested for as well. As a rule, these drugs are
not a good choice for patients who have a history of cancer
and of course are contraindicated in patients actively being
treated for cancer. Having psoriasis itself actually increases
the risk of some types of lymphoma, taking biologic drugs may
or may not increase this risk. As a class, the TNF-alpha blocking drugs share several side effects and warnings beyond
serious infections and malignancy:

- Patients with a history of any sort of demyelinating
  disorder such as multiple sclerosis should not use
  TNF-alpha blocking drugs
- Those with congestive heart failure should not use
  these drugs.
- TNF-alpha blocking drugs have been linked to blood
  problems like pancytopenia (decrease in production

of all blood cell types) and aplastic anemia (complete loss of production of red blood cells). Routine blood tests should be done while taking these drugs and any problems such as fever, bleeding, bruising, and pallor (unusual paleness) should be reported immediately.

- No live vaccines should be taken while on TNF-alpha blockers (or any biologic for that matter).
- Autoimmune and lupus-like problems have been reported with these drugs.

For further details, consult your physician.

Monitoring for Drug Toxicity of Biologics as Recommended by the NPF

Baseline Blood Testing

If you are using or considering using a biologic drug for psoriasis, you probably wonder what type of monitoring is needed to safely use these drugs. While there is little evidence-based data telling us exactly how to monitor for these drugs, the National Psoriasis Foundation has published their consensus committee's report on how they think the drugs should be monitored. Such reports are helpful guidelines but are not etched in stone - other groups may have other guidelines or recommendations which differ from these.

All the biologics require a baseline chemistry panel consisting of labs which look at liver and kidney function. They all require a complete blood count with platelets.

What is Psoriasis?

Tuberculosis Testing

All the biologic drugs affect the immune system, therefore there is concern that serious infections may occur more commonly with their use. Tuberculosis is a serious infection which may lie dormant for many years, then become reactivated when the immune system is hindered by biologic drug use. For this reason, routine checking for prior TB exposure with a skin test called the PPD (purified protein derivative) is suggested.

ANA Testing at Baseline

The ANA test is a screening test for lupus and lupus-like diseases. The TNF-alpha blocking biologics (Humira, Enbrel and Remicade) have all been associated with positive ANA tests and lupus-like syndromes. For this reason, a minority of doctors recommend testing for positive ANA before using these drugs. However, having a positive ANA is not an absolute contra-indication (reason to not use)these drugs. Also, it is fairly common for the ANA test to become positive while on these drugs, but the meaning or significance of this change is not fully understood.

Periodic Monitoring

Once baseline evaluation is done and a biologic drug started, periodic re-testing is done to monitor for side effects. The TNF-alpha blocking drugs (Humira, Enbrel and Remicade) require a repeat CBC and blood chemistry panel every 2-6 months while under treatment.

Patients on biologic drugs should undergo annual PPD testing to look for exposure to TB while undergoing treatment.

What are the Side Effects of Biologic Drugs for Psoriasis?

Question: What are the Side Effects of Biologic Drugs for Psoriasis?

Biologic drugs for psoriasis are highly effective. Since these drugs touch on sensitive systems such as the immune system, their use may result in certain side effects. This should be considered when choosing or using these medications for treatment of psoriasis.

Answer:

By and large, all biologics for psoriasis effect the immune system at some level. For this reason, the risk of serious infections are one of the possible side effects of these drugs. Less obvious to some patients is the role that the immune system plays in preventing the development of cancer.

There is at least a theoretical risk of malignancy with the use of these drugs for this reason. What most of the data shows to date is that the overall risk of malignancy with the use of biologic drugs parallels that seen in patients with psoriasis already. That is to say that the risk of malignancy in psoriasis or in psoriasis treated with biologic drugs is only very slightly increased, if at all, versus the general population.

There are also reports of abnormal blood tests while using these medications. Your doctor may feel it is appropriate to monitor blood work while you are on these medications

Because some of these drug may re-activate latent or hidden tuberculosis, it is recommended for some of the biologics that a pre-treatment test called a PPD is performed to see if the

What is Psoriasis?

patient being considered for those biologics has been exposed to tuberculosis. Talk to your doctor about the need for a TB test prior to using biologics.

Rarely, there have been reports of demyelinating disorders such as multiple sclerosis occurring with the use of TNF alpha blocking biologics. It is believed that, rather than causing MS, TNF alpha blockers may unmask or expose hidden MS in those prone to the disease.

Can Biologic Drugs Cause Psoriasis?

Question: Can Biologic Drugs Cause Psoriasis?
Biologic drugs are now being commonly used to treat moderate to severe psoriasis. With tens of thousands of patients being treated with these drugs, some more unusual effects have been noted. Can the same powerful biologic drugs we use to treat psoriasis actually make the disease break out?

Answer:
Although it seems counterintuitive, there are many reported cases of patients developing psoriasis while taking anti-TNF alpha biologic drugs -- the same drugs often prescribed to *treat* the skin condition.

Let's dig into the data on the patients who've experienced this perplexing result: Most of them were being treated with these drugs for conditions other than psoriasis, including arthritis or inflammatory bowel disease. A few were actually being treated for psoriasis, but developed new lesions or a change to a more serious form of psoriasis while on the drugs.

What is Psoriasis?

So, a patient would no longer have this side effect if her doctor took her off of the biologic drug, right?

It's not that simple. In some cases, the psoriasis went away if the anti-TNF drug was discontinued, but additional treatment for the newly-triggered psoriasis was needed in others.

That last part hints that perhaps some of these patients were destined for this result whether they used the drug or not.

Regardless of the medication you are taking, it's important that you take note of any side effects or changes you are experiencing and raise them to your doctor. Never stop biologic drugs abruptly unless you doctor tells you to. Sometimes a simple switch to the medication you are taking can be made -- but your physician won't know there's a need for it unless you raise your hand. And if it turns out that the drug's not to blame, your doctor will have a jump start on investigating what other health concerns may be developing.

Histoplasmosis - A Rare Fungal Infection Associated with Biologic Drugs

Histoplasmosis is a rare fungal infection more commonly seen in people with poorly functioning immune systems such as people with AIDS, those receiving strong chemotherapy and those taking other medications which can alter immune function. Typically, histoplasmosis causes flu-like symptoms with cough and in some patients skin lesions such as ulcerations. Because it is an uncommon ailment, diagnosis is often delayed allowing the disease to progress to an advanced state.

What is Psoriasis?

In September 2008, the FDA ordered the makers of 4 biologic drugs to include a specific warning about the increased risk of histoplasmosis in patients taking these drugs. The drugs included in the warning are Enbrel, Remicade, Humira and Cimzia (the first three are used for both arthritis and psoriasis, the last one is used for Crohn's disease). So far, 240 cases of histoplasmosis have been diagnosed in patients using these drugs. Of these patients, at least 21 had a delayed diagosis and 12 of them died. Even with timely diagnosis the disease is dangerous: 45 people out of the 240 infected died.

What does this mean for you?
If you are currently being treated with one of these biologic drugs and you develop symptoms such as persistent fever, cough, shortness of breath and fatigue, you should contact you doctor and perhaps express your concerns about the possibility of histoplasmosis so that this diagnosis will not be overlooked.

Humira (Adalimumab)

Convenience of Twice Monthly Injections:
Humira (adalimumab) is Abbott's biologic for psoriatic arthritis and rheumatoid arthritis. Approval for treatment of psoriasis was granted in the first quarter of 2008.

Who Should Take This Drug?:
Patients with psoriatic arthritis and patients with extensive plaque psoriasis) whose symptoms may have not improved with the more commonly used Enbrel (Etanercept), or who need the convenience of twice-monthly dosing.

What is Psoriasis?

Which Patients Should Avoid This Drug?:
Patients with severe infections, including tuberculosis or hepatitis B, and possibly those patients allergic to rubber or latex. Also, those people with multiple sclerosis and related neurological conditions, heart failure, upcoming vaccination or surgery, or who are pregnant or breastfeeding.

How is this Drug Used?:
Humira is self-injected under the skin once every two weeks.

What are the Side Effects of Humira?:
More common side effects include reactions at the site of injection (redness, rash, swelling, itching or bruising) as well as headache, nausea and upper respiratory tract infections. All drugs of this class (TNF alpha blockers) have a poorly defined increased risk of serious infection, neurological problems, and heart failure which needs to be balanced against their superior effectiveness in treating psoriasis.

Enbrel (Etanercept)

Effectiveness Combined with Impressive Safety Record: Enbrel (etanercept) was one of the first biologics. It was introduced for rheumatoid arthritis in 1998. In 2002, it was approved for use in psoriatic arthritis and finally, for plaque type psoriasis in 2004.

Who Should Take This Drug?: Enbrel is approved for adults with plaque type psoriasis or psoriatic arthritis. It is also approved for rheumatoid arthritis in adults and children as young as 4 -- a testament of sorts to is overall safety.

Which Patients Should Avoid This Drug?: Patients with serious infections, tuberculosis, hepatitis B or sepsis should avoid this drug. Caution should also be used in anyone with a demyelinating disorder (diseases such as multiple sclerosis, optic neuritis and others) as well as patients with a history of serious blood problems, such as low blood counts or aplastic anemia.

What are the Side Effects of Enbrel?: In psoriasis clinical trials, etanercept showed no higher incidence of serious adverse events, serious infections, TB or opportunistic infections than placebo.

Stelara- A Biologic with Quarterly Dosing

What is it:
Stelara is a biologic drug developed by Centocor (a drug company) that blocks two natural chemicals involved in psoriasis: IL12 and IL 23. Centocor is also the maker of Remicade (Infliximab) for psoriasis.

How Well Does It Work:
Stelara was effective and very lasting in a phase III clinical trial. After just two doses, 76% of patients in the high-dose part of the study achieved PASI 75 at week 12. Seventy-nine of these patients maintained PASI 75 at 28 weeks with three doses of drug. The drug appears to wear off slowly over time without a "rebound" or flare as seen with discontinuation of other treatments. The rates of adverse events was similar for drug vs. placebo. After an initial two closely-spaced doses, additional dosing is planned to be only once every 12 weeks making this in essence a quarterly drug. More recent data showed that patients on Stelara were more likely to experience cardiac problems than those on TNF-alpha blocking drugs, however the exact significance of this is not yet known.

What is Psoriasis?

Further Reading:

Stelara vs. Enbrel

Here's a relatively rare event: a true head-to-head study comparing two rival drugs. Usually doctors have to compare the results of one study with the results of another study and try to decide if one drug is better than another. In this study, Johnson and Johnson compared Stelara with the reigning champ, Enbrel. They found that nearly twice as many high-dose Stelara patients reached a PASI 90 score than enbrel patients. Is Stelara the end for Enbrel? Not really. Enbrel trumps Stelara by being able to treat not just psoriasis but psoriatic arthritis as well.

More on Enbrel (etanercept)

In a study out of Korea, Enbrel was effective in moderate psoriasis at about half the doses usually used in the US. The study investigators based their study on the notion that even moderate psoriasis would be as emotionally stressful for Asians as severe psoriasis is for Caucasians as the incidence and severity of psoriasis as well as the understanding of psoriasis in the Asian population is less. Using smaller doses obviously saves a lot of money for this expensive drug.

And if you're currently on Enbrel and not getting the results you expected, adding methotrexate to your program may improve your psoriasis, even if methotrexate taken alone in the past did not work well for you. Seems the combination provides a synergistic effect.

Enbrel for the "Heartbreak of Psoriasis"

In a study presented at the 17th European Academy of Dermatology and Venereology, Enbrel (etanercept) was shown to improve both depression and anxiety in psoriasis patients. The degree of improvement correlated with the degree of improvement in the patients' skin. The idea of psoriasis being associated with depression is not a new one. What we don't know yet, is whether or not etanercept is improving depression by treating psoriasis, or does it have an anti-depressant effect all its own?

Humira Reduces C-reactive Protein

A recent study showed that Humira when given to patients with psoriasis and elevated C-reactive protein normalized the levels of the C-reactive protein. I find this interesting with all the current attention on psoriasis increasing risk of myocardial infarction and the role of C-reactive protein as a marker of elevated risk of myocardial infection as well. Perhaps then we should be looking at treating psoriasis in the broader sense ie: not just the skin rash, but reducing the risk of associated illnesses through the use of drugs like Humira.

Enbrel Reduces C-Reactive Protein

A new study has shown that Enbrel (etanercept) given to patients with psoriasis and or psoriatic arthritis reduced C-Reactive Protein, a marker for inflammation. CRP is also believed to play a role in acute myocardial infarction. It is not clear yet whether or not Enbrel reduces the risk of AMI, but rheumatologist treating rhematoid arthritis with Enbrel seem to think so.

Section 12

Quality of Life and Psoriasis Treatment - Why PASI Scores Matter

Psoriasis definitely affects the health-related quality of life (HRQoL) of those suffering from this disease. Various measure of HRQoL include the Koo-Mentor Instrument among others.

The degree to which psoriasis affects a patient's HRQoL does not clearly correlate with their baseline level of disease. Some patients cope better than others. What does correlate well is the improvement of HRQoL seen with improvement in PASI score during treatment. In order to see a large impact in HRQoL, a large improvment in PASI score, such as PASI 75 or greater must be achieved. What this means is that a 75% reduction in psoriasis severity is sort of a threshold below which large changes in a patient's health-related quality of life are less likely. Many biologic drugs are indeed capable of achieving this level of improvement especially newer drugs such as Stelara.

Question: Can I Get a Tattoo if I Have Psoriasis?

Tattoos are popular in western culture and psoriasis is relatively common. Can people with psoriasis get tattoos or will doing so cause a flare up of their condition?

What is Psoriasis?

Answer:

Any trauma to the skin in a patient with psoriasis can cause the typical plaques of psoriasis to develop, a phenomenon known as the Koebner response. So can getting a tattoo cause the Koebner response? The answer is an unequivocal: *yes*. In fact, Dr. Koebner himself reported the development of psoriasis in a tattoo way back in 1872.

That being said, there are many people with psoriasis who can get tattoos without any problems. First decide: Is the tattoo really necessary? Then speak with your doctor about the risks involved. If a plaque of psoriasis develops due to a tattoo, it can likely be treated. Also, psoriasis doesn't always immediately develop right after getting a tattoo -- it may show up years later in the same spot as the tattoo.

How Can I Understand Clinical Trials?

 Question: How Can I Understand Clinical Trials?
Clinical trials are required to document that a drug works (and to get an idea of safety and side effects as well). What goes into the design of a clinical trial and what does it mean?

Answer:
Scientists use clinical trials to more or less prove that a certain drug, procedure or device works. By proof is meant that (statistically speaking) if the trial was repeated again and again, there is a very high likelihood that the results would be the same almost every time.

Numbers, such as an improvement in psoriasis PASI scores, are often reported with a "p-value" quoted, for example:

p<0.001. What this tells us is that the likelihood of that beneficial result being found and erroneously reported when in fact the drug had no effect is very small, less than 1 in 1,000. When "p-values" are small, the study has *statistical significance*. Larger studies with more patients and low p-values have more *power* and may carry more weight or believability than smaller trials with equally low and significant p-values.

Measuring results, which is often done by human observers, can result in bias that makes results less believable. In order to try and remove bias, trials can be blinded to keep participants and observers from knowing if they are getting the treatment or not. A trial where neither party knows whose getting active treatment and where a mock or placebo treatment is given is called a double-blind, placebo-controlled trial.

Another trial design often used is a cross-over trial, during which one group of patients is treated with a sequence of treatments, separated in time, and the response to the different treatments is compared.

What is a PASI Score?

Question: What is a PASI Score?
When reading about a new treatment, the results in the form of the PASI score are often quoted. What does this mean?

Answer:
The PASI score stands for Psoriasis Area and Severity Index. This tool allows researchers to put an objective number on what would otherwise be a very subjective idea: how bad is a person's psoriasis. To make up the score, the three features of a psoriatic plaque (redness) scaling and thickness are each as-

What is Psoriasis?

signed a number from 0 to 4 with 4 being worst. Then the extent of involvement of each region of the body is scored from 0 to 6. Adding up the scores give a range of 0 to 72.

Many studies quote the improvement seen in the PASI score over time as a measure of a drug's effectiveness. For example, they may note that a certain proportion of patients experienced a 75% reduction in their PASI scores over a 12-week treatment period and report this as a percentage of people achieving "PASI 75."

PASI scores are seldom used in clinical practice, although more fastidious doctors or those working at university-based clinics or specialized psoriasis treatment centers may routinely use this tool to follow their patients' progress.

Can Psoriasis of the Nails be Treated?

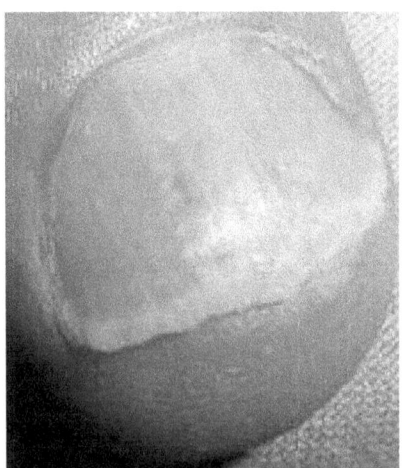

nail pitting ©New Paradigm Dermatology, PL

Question: Can Psoriasis of the Nails be Treated?

What is Psoriasis?

Psoriasis of the nails can cause lifting, thickening, pitting and other changes. Treatment can be difficult but worthwhile when healthy nails finally appear.

Answer: Nail psoriasis is difficult to treat: It takes about 5 months to grow a fingernail, and treatment needs to be maintained the entire time. The only topical medication that has substantial research backing its usefulness in treating nail psoriasis is tazarotene[1]. When this fails, intralesional steroids (injections directly into the root of the nail) may help improve the condition. This may sound unpleasant, but the procedure is quick and easy to do. Healthy nails usually reappear after a series of three monthly injections.

Further Reading:

Is Psoriasis More Common than Previously Thought?
Most sources say that psoriasis affects 2% of the Western population. But a study in the Journal of the American Academy of Dermatology indicates that there may be many more people suffering from psoriasis than previously thought. Looking at patients with lower socioeconomic status revealed that many more patients had psoriasis that was not diagnosed. As a result, it may be that up to 5% of people has psoriasis, just that many have not been "officially" diagnosed with the disease.

Is it Psoriasis, Nail Fungus, or Both?
Those thick, yellow and brittle nails may be due to psoriasis, but did you know that psoriatic nails are actually more prone to fungal infection than healthy nails? That's to say that you can easily have both conditions affecting your nails at the same time. Just treating the fungal infection is unlikely to provide significant cosmetic benefit if the psoriasis remains

untreated, so it may be necessary to treat both, either concurrently or sequentially.

Psoriasis Patients "Get Used to It" (that look of disgust)
A lot goes on subconsiously when we look at someone and when we notice them looking at us. Even the expression on their face is a tell or a signal of their opinion of us at that time.

It seems that when we look at something with disapproval, we put on a special face that signals disgust - and that signals is received. Apparently psoriasis patients are used to getting this signal. So used to it that they no longer respond to it as strongly as others.

University of Manchester docs using a functional MRI scan looked at that part of the brain (the insula) which is involved in interpreting these signals. Psoriasis patients demonstrated a reduced response to the digsust signal. This was felt to be a learned response which helps psoriasis patients to cope with their disease, and is in essence a part of living with psoriasis.

What is Psoriasis?

www.ingramcontent.com/pod-product-compliance
Lightning Source LLC
Chambersburg PA
CBHW072311290526

45794CB00002B/616